Intermittent Fasting for Women

The COMPLETE Beginner's Guide to BURNING FAT, Heal Your BODY and Increase ENERGY through Keto Diet, Fasting and Autophagy. How to Do it Right and AVOID COMMON MISTAKES

Table of Content

Foreword

Whether we like it or not, obesity is a worldwide phenomenon which is spreading like wildfire amongst men and women all over the world, but especially in the Western world. There are a few factors which are known to boost obesity, like the food type consumed, the overall lifestyle and stress. Also, there are too many situations when obesity is not experienced just by itself, and it comes along with other diseases and medical conditions, like diabetes, heart, liver or kidney diseases and sometimes even cancer.

The food we eat is causing most of the health problems known to man these days, as it has plenty of carbohydrates and almost none other macronutrients. As it turns out, we can't live just on carbs, as we also need proteins, lipids (fats), and minerals and vitamins. Most of the food we consume today is processed, and I'm not referring just to fast food, I'm also referring to most of the food sold in supermarkets. If the food comes with a package and has very strange ingredients, then that food is processed. When checking the label for ingredients, you will also notice the nutritional value of it. Most of the processed food is very high in sugar or salt, while the protein or fat content is very low. That's why this kind of food has little to no nutritional value, yet it has too many calories. Therefore, processed food is more calorie dense than nutrient dense.

Sugar is a type of carbohydrate, which is very common in the food we eat. It's also one of the most harmful substances the human body can encounter. This substance is responsible for more deaths than drugs, alcohol or cigarettes. Governments have tried to make the consumers aware of the consequences of sugar consumption by marking the labels of processed food with different colors if the sugar level of the food or drink is above or normal compared to the daily recommended dosage. Some of them have even implemented a sugar tax imposed on soft drinks, juices or other products with very high levels of sugar.

Sugar contains glucose, which under most circumstances is the most used energy source for the body. However, energy is not produced by eating carbs, instead is generated by burning glucose. But this process only happens if the body engages in physical activity, and unfortunately eating carbs gets you more tired than energized. Just think about it! You consume plenty of carbs, so you have high levels of glucose. The glucose should be used by the body to generate energy, but this only happens when the body is active. If the glucose is not used, it will get stored in your blood, raising the insulin and high blood level. Sound familiar? This is how diabetes starts. However, processed food gives you a satiety feeling for a short period of time, so you will be craving more carbs from processed food in no time. More food means more calories and also more glucose. So not only will you be storing glucose, but you will also be storing fat, as you don't give the body the chance to burn calories and fat tissue. You are constantly feeding the body with this low-quality food, which requires higher levels of consumption. When you are eating that many calories, and you are not involved in physical activity, guess what? You will start to gain weight and unless you are changing what you eat and start to exercise, you will not be able to stop and reverse the weight gaining process.

Cutting down on carbs is the right solution when it comes to nutrition. But what exactly you can eat instead? The answer is simple. Try to replace them with healthy fats. As you change the energy source of your body, from glucose to fats, the body will start using fats, therefore burning them. This is how you can set the body to run on fats and to decrease the fat tissue, thus reversing not only obesity, but also some other diseases and medical conditions as well.

Physical activity is what triggers the fat burning process if all the available glucose is burned and the body is using a different type of fuel, which can be found in the fat tissue, but also in high-fat meals. If we analyze the modern lifestyle, we can notice that there is little time to eat and even less time to exercise, as the modern job requires plenty of tasks to be done during the day and tight deadlines. This means more hours spent at work, less time to eat well and work out, and even less time to sleep. It also comes with plenty of stress. Remember, stress is a psychological condition which favors the consumption of processed food and snacks, so more calories. Therefore, it's fair to say that stress encourages obesity.

Women are more and more preoccupied with their looks, so being overweight is definitely something that can bother them. They are more keen on watching their weight than men, however, they are willing to spend less time exercising. Instead, women like to focus on trying all kinds of diets, many of them that are too radical and have harmful effects on their health. Trying diets without consulting a physician or a nutritionist has become a popular trend. Plenty of these diets require more or fewer restrictions, some of them are very harsh and most people break them because they can't stick to them anymore, or they are not feeling very well after trying them. After quitting the diet, most people will return to normal eating habits and will start to regain weight quite fast. Therefore, women should look for the best-balanced diets and should stick to them for a very long time, transforming them into a lifestyle. This book can show you a few very healthy alternatives when it comes to losing weight.

Chapter 1: What Is Intermittent Fasting?

Nowadays, people are more and more exposed to processed foods, so there are higher chances of consuming a higher level of carbs (and therefore glucose). Since there are around 70% of the diseases known to man caused by processed food, people are trying to find a solution to this problem. Analyzing the eating habits of prehistoric humans, and even those from more recent ages, scientists have come with a solution, which was already implemented by some religious sects. This solution is called fasting, a very popular practice in religions like Islam, Judaism or even Christianity. The "pure" way to fast is to deprive yourself of food and water, with the intent of purifying your soul.

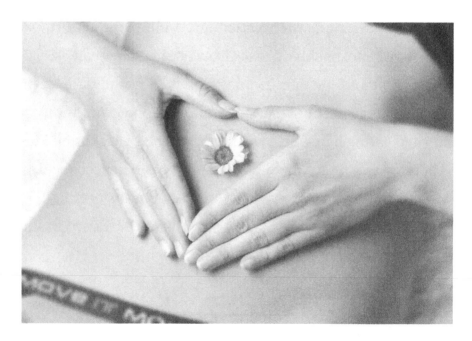

From a non-religious approach, fasting means the complete deprivation of food for a limited amount of time. Bearing this in mind, intermittent fasting (or IF for short) is an alternate cycle between feeding period and fasting period. There is no mention of what food you need to eat, so this procedure is more about scheduling your meals than what your meals include. The only thing you need to worry about is to sticking to the schedule. However, this doesn't mean that you can only eat fast food, or copious amounts of processed food, as one of the most important goals of this practice is to train your body to run on fats, not on glucose, and to favor the fat burning process. So, cutting down on carbs may be something very helpful when it comes to this diet.

Fasting doesn't mean the period between your meals of the day, as a period of 4 hours between meals is not considered fasting. Specialists would probably argue about what is the minimum period of time for fasting. Some would say between 12 and 14 hours, others would say at least 16 hours. However, when it comes to IF, you need to distinguish the difference between the fasting period and the fasted state. The first one is the period during which you are not consuming any calories at all, so you are not eating. The second term is more about a metabolic state during which the body starts to run on fats. The fasted state starts 12 hours after your last meal, after the glucose has been burned or processed, and the body can't seem to find other "fuel types" to use as energy. Switching to fats seems to be the obvious choice since glucose is no longer available. The energy from the fat tissue can only be released through the actions of ketones, molecules released by your liver specially designed to break through the fat cells. However, more details regarding ketones, ketosis and the keto-adaptation process can be found in the following chapters of this book.

Getting back to intermittent fasting, it's important to understand that the source of inspiration for it comes from history. Let's think about prehistoric humans and their lifestyle. In order to feed, these humans had to hunt, fish or pick fruits. Food wasn't always available, and nobody knew exactly when the next meal was planned to be. People were able to go for days without food. As a result, the prehistoric human was a lot stronger, faster and more agile than the modern-day human. Let's face it, the quality of food was a lot better back then, as everything was a natural (unlike today). However, as it turns out, fasting for a longer period can improve your concentration and can also increase the level of growth hormone. Therefore, fasting was not only very good for their muscle mass, but also for their focus. A more detailed approach on the benefits (and also the downsides) of intermittent fasting can be found in the chapter below. Food was not very available back then, and it required skill to procure it. Although it wasn't their intent, people were fasting on a regular basis back in the day. Having 3 meals each day was not possible, so they had a very different lifestyle than the one we have today. It was also a lot more active, as it involved running, climbing trees and possibly swimming, activities which are done today only by a few of us.

Some nutritionists would agree that intermittent fasting "is perhaps the oldest and most powerful dietary intervention imaginable."[1] IF is more about self-discipline, and less about starvation. If you "play your cards right", then your body will be able to resist starvation and you can go on fasting for a longer period. Control makes a difference in this case. Starvation may be caused by not having anything to eat (no control), whilst fasting is, in fact, a voluntary deprivation from food for different reasons, whether it's fat loss, overall health, or spiritual reasons. The purists would say that there is only one type of fast, the water fast. This is the most radical way of fasting, but there are also other ways, which are less harsh,

---

1 Fung, Jason, and Andreas Eenfeldt. "Intermittent Fasting for Beginners – The Complete Guide – Diet Doctor." *Diet Doctor*, 21 May 2019, www.dietdoctor.com/intermittent-fasting/.

and you will find more details about them in another chapter of this book.

Women are more sensitive when it comes to changes in their meal plan and the food they eat, but they should know that intermittent fasting is simply not for everyone. If they are breastfeeding, pregnant or underweight (also if they have an eating disorder such as anorexia), they shouldn't practice this way of eating. However, if they don't have any of these conditions, they are eligible for intermittent fasting, but still, they need to see a physician or a nutritionist first. If you are expecting unbelievable weight loss, then you will be most likely disappointed. This process is more about preparing the body for weight loss (in this case, fat burning) because it needs to be paired with physical exercise in order to be more effective.

It's said that intermittent fasting has 5 or 6 different stages, as seen below:

1) Ketosis - a metabolic state which should get activated 12 hours after your last meal. Ketone level is going up, and this favors the breaking down of fat tissue, thus releasing the energy stored in the fat cells. Let's say that you have the last meal at 6 pm, this means you should be entering the ketosis phase the next day at 6 am. The human brain is capable of using 60% of the glucose

whilst the body rests.[2] Ketones are starting to become the default fuel type for now.

2) Fat-burning mode - 18 hours after your last meal, the body runs now just on fats, as the ketones level is very high, so more ketones mean more fats burned.

3) Recycling old cells' components - a state which occurs 24 hours after your last meal. Not only these parts are being recycled, but also other misfolded or old proteins are being destroyed. These proteins can be associated with diseases like Parkinson and Alzheimer's. This phase is also known as *autophagy*.

4) The growth hormone level reaches a level which is 5 times higher than the one at the beginning of your fast. This happens after 48 hours of the fasting period, during which you didn't have any calories at all. This hormone is responsible for preserving your muscle mass but also can prevent fat tissue accumulation.

5) After 54 hours of fasting, the insulin level reaches unbelievably low levels. The lower your insulin level is,

---

2 Jarreau, Paige, and Essential Information. "The 5 Stages of Intermittent Fasting." *LIFE Apps | LIVE and LEARN*, 26 Feb. 2019, lifeapps.io/fasting/the-5-stages-of-intermittent-fasting/.

the more active it gets. Apparently, the best way to activate your insulin and let it determine how to do its job (regulating the blood sugar level, or lowering it) is to lower it. Well, this is what intermittent fasting does to the insulin level.

6) Recycling old immune cells and generating brand new ones. This phase happens after 72 hours of fasting.

Chapter 2: Benefits and Side Effects of Intermittent Fasting

There are plenty of diets out there, all promising you the impossible. Incredible weight loss, with no mention of any side effects. You are probably fed up with the "lose x pounds in 30 days, guaranteed" approach. Many of these diets are not backed up by science, or in other words, there is not any scientific research to prove these diets actually deliver what they promise. They focus only on the weight loss process, suggesting meal plans that are extremely radical in some cases.

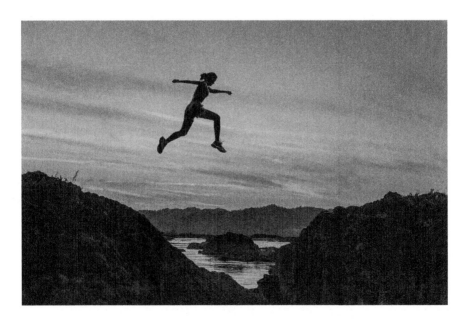

Diets mean nutrient deprivation in most cases, but they are plenty of cases when these diets have harmful effects on your health. Unlike other diets, focused on the weight loss process in an incredibly short amount of time, intermittent fasting is focusing more on your health, as nutritionists believe that health should be the most important factor, and only a healthy body can have a long and sustainable weight loss process. Unlike the other diets, which have a "hit and run" approach, IF is something for the long run and should be regarded as a way of life, not like a meal plan to be implemented for a few weeks. By checking out the benefits below, you can better understand why this process is so beneficial for your body.

The main benefits of intermittent fasting can be summarized in 8 points:

- eliminates precancerous and cancerous cells
- shifts easily into nutritional ketosis
- reduces the fat tissue
- enhances the gene expression for health span and longevity
- induces autophagy and the apoptotic cellular repair or cleaning
- improves your insulin sensitivity
- reduces inflammation and oxidative stress
- increases neuroprotection and cognitive effects

To expand on the benefits of this practice, intermittent fasting can have positive impacts over the fat loss process, disease prevention, anti-aging, therapeutic benefits (psychological, spiritual and physical), mental performance, physical fitness (improved metabolism, wind, and endurance, the great effect over bodybuilding).

Intermittent Fasting for the Weight Loss Process

As you restrain yourself from eating, the body will no longer have available glucose to use in order to produce energy. Therefore, it will use ketones to break the fat tissue open and release the energy stored in there. This is how the body will burn your existing fat in order to generate energy. When it comes to diets, they are not designed for the long run, and as soon as you break the diet, you will start gaining weight again. Intermittent fasting is something that you can try for a lifetime because it is easy to stick to it, and it doesn't involve any special meal plan. So, you can still eat your favorite foods, as long as you schedule your meals, allowing a smaller eating window and a longer fasting period. IF induces ketosis and eventually autophagy, which will definitely mean reducing the fat reserves.

Intermittent Fasting for Preventing Diseases

What if you found out that intermittent fasting is, in fact, a cure for several different diseases and medical conditions? You would definitely become more interested in this process. There are a few studies that show the beneficial effects IF has on your health. A study published in the *World Journal of Diabetes* has shown that patients with type 2 diabetes on short-term daily intermittent fasting experience a lower body weight, but also a better variability of post-meal glucose.

Other benefits this diet has are:

- enhances the markers of stress resistance
- reduces the blood pressure and inflammation
- better lipid levels and glucose circulation, which may lead to a lower risk of cardiovascular disease, neurological diseases like Parkinson's and Alzheimer's, and also cancer

Intermittent Fasting for the Anti-Aging Process

The modern-day lifestyle includes too much stress and is too sedentary. Whether we like it or not, these factors have a great contribution to the aging process. You are probably wondering what intermittent fasting can do the slow down this process, as we all know that it can't be stopped. IF is not "the fountain of youth" and it will not grant you immortality, but it can still lower the blood pressure and reduce oxidative damage, enhance your insulin sensitivity and reduce your fat mass. Coincidence or not, all of these are factors are known to improve your health and longevity. Intermittent fasting is one of the triggering factors of autophagy, a process known for destroying and replacing old cell parts with new ones, at any level within your body. Such a process can slow down the aging process.

Intermittent Fasting Practiced for Therapeutic Benefits

When it comes to therapeutic benefits, the most important ones are physical, spiritual and psychological. In terms of **physical benefits**, intermittent fasting is a powerful cure for diabetes, but it can also prove to be very useful for reducing seizure-related brain damage and seizures themselves, but also for improving the symptoms of arthritis. This practice also has a spiritual value, as it's widely practiced for religious purposes across the globe. Although fasting is regarded as penance by some practitioners, it's also a practice for purifying your body and soul (according to the religious approach).

Intermittent fasting is also about exercising control and will, over your body and your feelings. Achieving absolute control over your power and mind is a very powerful **psychological** benefit. You can ignore hunger, restrain yourself from eating for a certain period of time. In other words, IF is also associated with mind training and can also improve your self-esteem. A successful intermittent fasting regime can have very powerful effects from a psychological point of view. A study has shown that women practicing IF had amazing results in terms of senses of control, reward, pride, and achievement.

Intermittent Fasting for Better Mental Performance

IF also enhances the cognitive function and also is very useful when it comes to boosting your brain power. There are several factors of intermittent fasting which can support this claim. First of all, it boosts the level of brain-derived neurotrophic factor (also known as BDNF), which is a protein in your brain that can interact with the parts of your brain responsible for controlling cognitive and memory functions as well as learning. BDNF can even protect and stimulate the growth of new brain cells. Through IF, you will enter the ketogenic state, during which your body turn fat into energy, by using ketones. Ketones can also feed your brain, and therefore improve your mental acuity, productivity, and energy.

Intermittent Fasting for an Improved Physical Fitness

This process influences not only your brain but also your digestive system. By setting a small feeding window and a larger fasting period, you will encourage the proper digestion of food. This leads to a proportional and healthy daily intake of food and calories. The more you get used to this process, the less you will experience hunger. If you are worried about slowing your metabolism, think again! IF *enhances* your metabolism, it makes metabolism more flexible, as the body has now the capability to run on glucose or fats for energy, in a very effective way. In other words, intermittent fasting leads to better metabolism.

Oxygen use during exercise is a crucial part of the success of your training. You simply can't have performance without adjusting your breathing habits during workouts. VO2 max represents the maximum amount of oxygen your body can use per minute or per kilogram of body weight. In popular terms, VO2 max is also referred to as "wind". The more oxygen you use, the better you will be able to perform. Top athletes can have twice the VO2 level of those without any training. A study focused on the VO2 levels of a fasted group (they just skipped breakfast) and a non-fasted group (they had breakfast an hour before). For both groups, the VO2 level was at 3.5 L/min at the beginning, and after the study, the level showed a significant increase of "wind" for the fasting group (9.7%), compared to just 2.5% increase in the case of those with breakfast.

Intermittent Fasting for Bodybuilding

Having a narrow feeding window automatically mean fewer meals, so you can concentrate the daily calorie intake into just 1-2 consistent meals. Bodybuilders find this approach a lot more pleasing than having the same calorie consumption split into 5 or 6 different meals throughout the day. It's said that you need a specific amount of proteins just to maintain your muscle mass. However, muscle mass can be also maintained through intermittent fasting, a process which doesn't focus specifically on protein intake. Remember, the growth hormone reaches unbelievable levels after 48 hours of fasting, so you can easily maintain your muscles without eating many proteins, or having protein bars or shakes.

As you already know, nothing is perfect and intermittent fasting is no exception. There are a few **side effects** that you need to worry about, like:

- **hunger** is perhaps the most common side effect of this way of eating, but the more you get used to IF, the less hunger you will feel
- beware of **constipation,** as when you eat less, you will not have to go to the toilet very often, so you can feel constipated at the beginning
- **headaches** should be expected when fasting. Food deprivation is a direct cause of these headaches. However, controlling your hunger and getting used to fasting, will be the best weapon to fight against these headaches
- during intermittent fasting, you might experience muscle cramps, heartburn, and dizziness
- in the case of athletic women, or those with very low body fat percentage, intermittent fasting may lead to a higher risk of irregular periods and lower chances of conception (so it reduces fertility for these women)

Chapter 3: Types of Intermittent Fasting

There are several intermittent fasting programs you can choose from according to your needs and goals you want to achieve. Burning fats seems to be one of the main goals of IF, regardless of the program you choose.

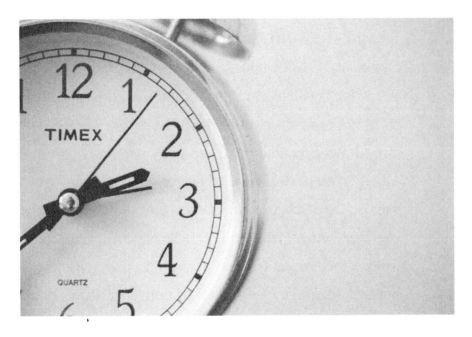

Considering the fasting period you are trying to set, or the reduction of calories, there are a few fasting programs which are worth to be mentioned.

1) **The Leangains Program** (also known as the 16/8 hours fast) is a daily fasting program which allows the body plenty of time to burn fats. It splits the day into 2 periods: 8 hours of feeding and 16 hours of fasting. The

16/8 hours fast program is a program which can be easily practiced by most of the women out there, unless they have a special medical condition or they are pregnant, trying to conceive a baby or have an eating disorder. It usually involves skipping one important meal of the day, and most nutritionists would suggest skipping breakfast. Considering breakfast the most important meal of the day is a myth, as in this case, you can easily skip breakfast and let your body burn fats. Scientists believe that the body goes into the fasted state 12 hours after your last meal. In this state, glucose is no longer available, so the body will start to run on fats. It's the perfect time to exercise. If you have the last meal at 6 pm, then you will start the fasted state at 6 am the next day. You can choose several options for physical exercise, and if it's more intense than it's even better. Jogging, cycling, swimming, or intense gym training are perfect options for morning exercise which are guaranteed to burn fat. The 16 hour fasting period should be respected, and you shouldn't consume any calories during this period. Plus, at least 7 hours during this fasting period you should be asleep. The Leangains program involves setting up a few things like:

- when to start your feeding window, and how long should it last? Although the recommended time frame for the eating period is 8 hours, you can even go lower than that, for example having an eating period of 6 hours (the lower your feeding window is, the better for your body). You can start it at 10 am and finish it at 6 pm.

- the fasting period is very important, as it needs to be around 16 hours or more, and it should include your sleeping period as well. During these 16 hours, you need to avoid consuming any kind of calories, so you can only drink water.

- don't forget about physical exercise, as you need to establish when it's the best time to work out. All specialists would agree that intense training during the fasted state (more than 12 hours after your last meal) is the perfect time to work out, as your body will use only fats to generate energy.

Following this program is not an easy thing to do, in fact, it can be a bit of a challenge. However, to make sure you have very good results when implementing the Leangains program, make sure you respect the following tips:

- Make sure you consume enough proteins in the feeding window but don't try to compensate in one day if you had several days with lower protein intake.

- Working out is a must for this program.

- If you plan on consuming carbs, make sure you do it on the workout days, as you definitely want to burn the excess glucose.
- Focus on eating consistent meals (by consistent I mean nutrient-dense food, not calorie bombs with very low nutritional value) during the feeding period, and make sure you don't consume any calories during the fasting period (drink only water, don't eat anything, not even snacks).
- Since physical exercise is a part of this program, make sure you don't eat anything before the training, and have the most consistent meal of the day right after training.
- If you don't have any exercise planned for a specific day, you still need to have the first meal as the most consistent one of the day.

Whether you choose to have a feeding window of 6 or 8 hours is up to you. It's possible to squeeze all 3 main meals of the day in 8 hours, but in 6 hours it's impossible. Having a daily fasting process is very good for your body, as it can function at optimal parameters and also burn fat while doing it. This program is highly appreciated by bodybuilders. Although there is no mention of what kind of food you need to consume on a daily basis, it's recommended to cut down on carbs to make the program more effective. Lowering the eating window to just 4 hours per day takes intermittent fasting to a whole different level, called The Warrior Diet, but this program is too radical to be implemented by most women practically.

2) **The 24 hours fast**, or also known as *Eat Stop Eat*, is a program promoted by Brad Pilon, a fitness enthusiast. It means literally fasting for 24 hours, so no eating or snacking at all during this period. Just water. During this day you will allow plenty of time for the body to burn fats and experience all the other benefits of intermittent fasting. Therefore, you can have a normal feeding day, followed by 24 hours of fasting. If you have your last meal on Tuesday at 6pm, this means that you will have the next meal on Wednesday at 6pm. For better results, you can also work out on the fasting day and you can alternate the feeding days with fasting days for 2 or 3 times during any given week, depending on what you are trying to achieve. Not consuming anything in the fasting window doesn't mean you will have to compensate the calories in the feeding window. So make sure you don't overdo it when it comes to eating. Fasting for 24 hours or more shouldn't be a very tough practice, as in some religions fasting is a normal habit practiced widely. So if religious people can do it, so can you. Healthy food and physical exercise are also highly recommended, although this program doesn't mention

anything about the food you will need to eat or what kind of exercise you need to practice. Nutritionists recommend the day-long fast at least once a few weeks, however, there is nothing wrong with trying it on a more regular basis. The more often you use this type of fast, the more spectacular will be the results.

3) **The Alternate Day Fast (also known as 36/12 hour fast)** is a perfect example of fasting for a longer period, and unlike other intermittent fasting programs, this one was actually developed by a doctor, so this program can get extra credit for this specific reason. A famous nutritionist, Dr. James B. Johnson, is the person responsible for developing the Alternate Day Fast, as he wrote a book dedicated to this program, called "The Alternate Day Diet." The 36/12 hour fast involves having a 12-hour feeding period (which is quite normal, you can have all 3 main meals of the day during this feeding window), followed by 36 hours of fasting. It may sound long, but this fasting period is totally doable. However, to make sure the fasting period is easier to endure, make sure you have proper nutrient-dense food during the feeding period. Healthy fats and protein intake should be higher than the carb consumption. Since this program was not developed by a bodybuilder, it doesn't mention anywhere that you need to work out, however, to have better results you really should. This method is not that strict, as you can easily eat whatever

you like (as long as it's healthy) in the 12 hour eating window, and that's why it should be perfect for beginners.

You will need to follow a few simple rules like:

a) Make sure you fast for at least 36 hours
b) Eat normally during the 12 hours feeding period
c) Although you can eat anything you want, it's highly recommended to have nutrient-dense foods instead of calorie-dense ones

During this program, you will need to establish the feeding and fasting windows:

1) Establish your feeding period as 12 hours during a day. Let's say you have your first meal at 7 am and the last one at 7 pm on a Monday, so you can repeat the same feeding schedule 4 days during a week (Monday, Wednesday, Friday, Sunday);
2) Your fasting window is 36 hours and should start after the last meal. Therefore, in this case, it should start at 7 pm on Monday and should last until 7 am on Wednesday.

This program was already tested on people, and it delivered really interesting results. The Alternate Day Diet not only has effects on the weight loss process, but it also has effects on your health. Volunteers who tested this program "lost on average 8% of their body weight over an eight-week period and experienced benefits such as reduced inflammation improved insulin resistance and better cellular energy production".[3] It's no surprise that intermittent fasting programs are capable of lowering blood pressure and this one makes no exception. It can also be the right program to induce autophagy and to ease arthritis. Having 36 hours of "pure" fast can be a bit too radical, especially for women, that's why Dr. James B. Johnson considers that you can have a very small calorie intake in the fasting period, around 500 calories. The rule, in this case, would be to consume 20% of the normal calorie intake. That's why, from his point of view, feeding days are considered Up Days, whilst the fasting days are considered Down Days. The 20% rule in the Down Days can apply in the first 2 weeks, but from week 3 you can increase the calorie intake from 20% to 35%. You are probably wondering what are you allowed to consume during the Down Days, and fruits and smoothies are the right choices. In order to make the program more efficient, you will also have to eat healthy during the eating window. Therefore, eating keto or Mediterranean is the right thing to do. Food types or drinks like chicken, fish, turkey, fruits, vegetables, eggs white, oats,

----

3   Matus,   Mizpah.   *Alternate   Day   Diet*, www.freedieting.com/alternate-day-diet.

whole wheat bread, high-fiber cereal, pasta, Shirataki noodles, and red wine should definitely be in your diet. Working out can't do you any harm, even on the fasting days, so you can combine this program with training for better fat-burning results.

The Alternate Day Fast has plenty of advantages like:

- it doesn't come with restrictions in terms of food, however, it's highly recommended to eat healthily and include the food types mentioned above in your diet
- the method is simple enough and easy to follow it for a long period of time
- deprivation is not something you need to worry about, as you can eat whatever you like during the feeding period
- you can trust this program even more, as it was developed by a real doctor
- it looks like this method can improve conditions like asthma
- this method can improve the metabolism and extend the lifespan (just like any other intermittent fasting method)

However, there are some downsides to this method, as you can see below:

- there is a higher risk of experiencing fatigue, dizziness, and hunger in the first days of practicing this program
- the method as developed by Dr. James B. Johnson doesn't mention anything about physical exercise, probably just to point out the major role the program has in the fat-burning process
- if you have an eating disorder like anorexia, you definitely shouldn't try this program

The Alternate Day Fast allows you to consume calories in the fasting days, and it doesn't mention any training or working out during this program. However, this doesn't mean that it's forbidden to practice a bit of physical exercise. Some people may consider this program the easiest one out there, so perhaps when they are thinking about trying intermittent fasting, this can be the first program they can try. However, if you are pregnant, breastfeeding, or have an eating disorder, you may need to stay away from IF.

4) **Water Fasting** is the "purest" program when it comes to intermittent fasting, and it's also the most radical one. No matter how healthy you are, you shouldn't try this program without the support and supervision of a physician. This should be tried as a last resort if no other IF programs work,

or if you want to achieve faster results. Even though people can go for hundreds of days using just water, probably the perfect example is one of an obese man who managed to fast for 382 days (consuming just water and vitamins) and lose 276 pounds. You will need to keep in mind that this method deprives you of all nutrients, minerals, and vitamins that come from food, so you better have a really strong reason to try it. Water fasting is regarded as a very good program for detoxing and fat burning. It will definitely make your body switch to the metabolic state of ketosis, and then it will induce autophagy (more about autophagy in a future chapter). This program is definitely not for everyone, as it's the best example of fasting for a longer period. Having nothing to eat for several days (people might even try it more than a week) is not very comfortable. You will experience all the possible side effects of intermittent fasting with this program like fatigue, dizziness, and hunger, but you will maximize the benefits of fat burning, disease prevention and other benefits to your health and physical condition. Of course, the method doesn't mention any workout or any sort of training. You should only try working out if you feel up to it, as when you are not having anything to eat at all, you will lack the necessary nutrients and you will not have glucose or fat from which the body can extract the energy. The second day of water fasting is probably the hardest one, as you will feel most hungry during this day. It's important to set your mind and overcome this situation and move on with the fasting process. As long as the days go by, you will feel more comfortable fasting. It's also important to keep your mind occupied, and not to think about food. However, you don't have to exaggerate and fast for too many days. You should fast for as long as you feel capable, but only with the supervision of a physician. There is also an alternative to the water fast, which is a bit less radical. It's called juice or broth fasting. Whilst juice can have plenty of vitamins and is mostly made out of fruits, you should try juices made out of vegetables because fruits have a lot more sugar than veggies. The broth is a type of soup which can have some proteins and nutrients, and you can also put a bit of fat into it. The human body can last for a few days without water, and for plenty more days without food. However, too many days without food is definitely not something recommendable. That's why most doctors would not recommend water fasting for more than 72 hours. If you are thinking about trying intermittent fasting, then you definitely need to start with a method which is a lot easier, like the ones mentioned previously in this chapter. Fasting for a very long time doesn't necessarily mean that it will bring you better results than if you fast for 16, 20 or 24 hours. In terms of fat burning, you can have better results with trying the Leangains Program associated with intense training and healthy food (keto diet seems to be the best choice).

5) **Fast Mimicking or Fat Fasting** is a very interesting alternative fasting program. What if you can actually eat and still fast? This is the best question to ask yourself when you are thinking of trying this program. Intermittent fasting is a procedure designed to make your body run on fats, and therefore burn more fats. Let's face it, water fasting is not for everyone, just for a few. Other fasting programs may be already too harsh in terms of lowering the feeding window and expanding the fasting window, so you will spend more time in the fasting window, not eating anything. The worst part is that the fasting window is not limited to sleeping. There is actually a method of fasting which doesn't involve splitting your day into fasting and feeding windows, so you don't have to worry about that. You can consume fats (yes, that's correct) in order to lose weight. You are probably asking, how is this possible? The answer is very simple.

"Your body doesn't distinguish dietary fat from metabolizing dietary fat, and therefore remains in the fasted state. This gives you the benefits of fasting while allowing you the macro and micronutrients your body needs to get into ketosis and all the benefits from brain and body fueled by ketones".[4]

---

4 The A-Z of Intermittent Fasting: Everything You Need to Know. (n.d.). *Perfect Keto*, p. 18.

Sound interesting enough? Well, take a look below to find out more about the advantages and benefits:

- it improves and regenerates the immune system
- it suppresses the precancerous and cancerous cells
- it triggers autophagy
- it activates ketosis which will help with the fat burning process
- it lowers the C-reactive protein and the oxidative stress
- it enhances your gene expression, and therefore it increases your longevity
- it can help improve your healthy stem cells, regenerative markers and fasting glucose
- it boosts your mental performance and also BDNF (brain-derived neurotrophic factor), which is crucial for the survival and growth of the new brain neurons

Chapter 4: The Weight Loss Process

Weight loss is one of the main benefits of intermittent fasting, regardless of the program you use. Everyone likes to lose some weight, especially if they are overweight, but do they want to lose muscle mass, or do they want to burn fat? Most would say that they want to burn fat, as fat is not aesthetically pleasing, and can also lead to health issues. However, if you are expecting miracles from any IF programs in terms of fat loss, think again! This lifestyle prepares the body to burn fats, but physical exercise is what enhances the fat burning process. Intermittent fasting is able to switch the default "fuel type" of the body from glucose to fat, so every activity that you do will break down the fat tissue and release the energy stored in there.

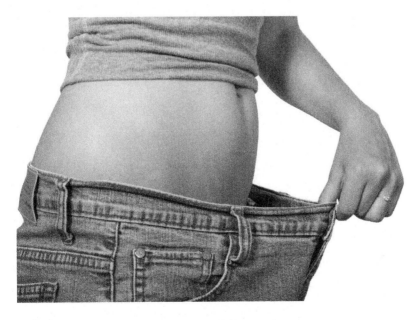

When it comes to the fat burning process, you really have to understand the term *ketosis*, which is a metabolic state during which the ketone body levels are going high and the insulin level is going low. Insulin is something that we are all aware of, but what about ketones? They are a class of organic compounds capable of breaking down the fat tissues in order to release the energy stored within them. A normal diet will get your body fed using glucose, which the body will need to burn in order to produce energy. Glucose can mostly be found in carbs, but they are also found in proteins. It's highly unlikely to burn all the glucose you consume, though, especially when the body is not engaged in physical activity. If the glucose is not consumed it gets stored in your blood and therefore it raises the blood sugar level. Not consuming carbs (rich in glucose), and even not consuming anything at all, will lower the insulin level and will raise the levels of ketones.

Through intermittent fasting, the body can enter ketosis 12 hours after your last meal. At this point, the body can't find any glucose available to use, so it's starting to look for alternative energy sources. The ketone bodies are multiplying, and they will help the body burn fat tissue to release the energy stored there.

If ketosis is a metabolic state during which the insulin, blood sugar and ketones bodies are all getting at an appropriate level, the keto-adaptation process is somewhat different, as it trains your body to run on ketones and fat as the default source of energy. So you don't have to rely on glucose as your energy source, you can instead use your existing stored fat or dietary fat (by dietary fat we mean the fats you eat through your meal plan, low-carb-high-fat [LCHF] diets are recommended). You can reach the keto-adaptation process through intermittent fasting when your body will use the energy stored in your fat reserves, but you can also induce it through nutritional ketosis (the keto diet is what can get you in this phase). "To become keto-adapted, you have to go through a period of being in ketosis where your liver's enzymes and metabolic processes change so you could have the ability to burn fat for fuel, but it's not necessary to be in ketosis all the time to maintain keto adaptation. You can briefly dip in and out of the ketosis for a day or two without fully losing it."[5]

Intermittent fasting is a process that can help you lose weight, mostly in terms of fat, but it doesn't mean that it will work miracles on you. It's not the kind of program to promise you will lose 10-20 pounds per week. Any diet promising you this is either unhealthy or just lying to get you on board. IF is instead one of the healthiest and most sustainable ways to lose

5 Land, S. (2018). *Metabolic autophagy*. Independently Published, p. 285-286

weight, as you can use this program for a very long time, while enjoying plenty of health benefits yourself, during which time you will slowly notice yourself losing some pounds. In the case of other diets, the more drastic the diet is, the more pounds you lose, but the more likely is for you to quit it soon and start gaining pounds immediately. Intermittent fasting is a program you can stick to, which encourage you to lose weight in a natural way. It's more of a lifestyle, which means that by following this way of eating you will not gain weight, but you will slowly lose weight, without having to cut out your favorite types of food.

Another very important aspect of IF is physical exercise, as it can make the difference between a very moderate weight loss (in terms of fat burn) and a very visible one. HIIT (High-Intensity Interval Training) can be the most effective for people to lose weight. It requires training very intensely with heavy weights and having just a few seconds as a break between exercises. By repeating the exercises, people feel their body burn fat and gain tone. However, this is something that isn't suitable for all women, so cardio and endurance exercises are recommended for those who are not suited to HIIT. Don't let the body rest too much, because this is how you will be able to burn fats. Having just 30 seconds of break time between exercises may be the ideal way to work out. This applies if you are going to the gym, you can also try some other forms of physical exercises, like jogging and swimming, or even cycling. Doing some ab exercises, squats, pushups and other physical exercises which can be done from home is also highly recommended. Exercising during the fasting period may be the best way to burn fats, as you will force your body to activate the ketones and break down the fat tissue for some fats.

If you are consuming dietary fat, the body will first consume it first, and only then switch to your stored fat. The transition is more smoothly than having glucose and then switching to the fat reserves, as your ketones are already very active in this case and it will not take too much time to switch the "fuel type" from glucose to fat. You can compare your body to a car, and the fat your body uses as an energy source with "biofuel."

To sum up, intermittent fasting can prepare your body for the fat-burning process, but the real fat burn is happening through physical exercise. By setting your body to run on fats, this will maximize the effects of the fat-burning process through physical exercise, as every bit of energy comes from fat. That's why exercising and fasting practiced more frequently can have better results in terms of weight loss than just doing fasting alone. Remember, your body needs to be in a keto-adapted state in order to burn fats very efficiently, and intermittent fasting can help you achieve this state, but especially in combination with a keto diet. More details on the keto diet can be found in a future chapter.

Chapter 5: Autophagy

The term autophagy can trace its roots to Ancient Greece and is the joining of two notions: "auto" (which means self) and "phagein" (which means to eat), therefore, in common words, autophagy means to eat oneself. A more detailed definition of this term can show us that is a mechanism used to get rid of old and damaged cell parts like cells membranes, organelles, and proteins. This can happen when the body lacks the energy to preserve the damaged and old cell machinery (which is composed of different cells parts mentioned above).

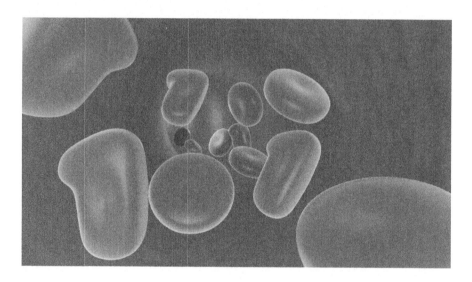

In other words, autophagy degrades and recycles all sorts of cellular parts, but it shouldn't be confused with apoptosis, which is the process of scheduling cell death. Although it sounds a bit cruel, apoptosis is exactly like an old car which is not working anymore, so you will need to dispose of the old and not-functioning parts. Apoptosis gets rid of the cells and replaces them with new ones. Autophagy basically does the same thing, but at a subcellular level.

The first autophagy studies were conducted on yeast, and the progress on this particular field of expertise also led to a Nobel Prize in October 2016. Dr. Yoshinori Ohsumi won the Nobel Prize in Physiology or Medicine for his "discoveries of the mechanisms for autophagy." However, autophagy is not present just in yeast, it's present in every living organism, even in the human body.

Since we already covered what autophagy is, you are probably wondering what can trigger it. "Autophagy, a cellular cleaning process, gets activated in response to certain types of metabolic stress, including nutrient deprivation, growth factor depletion, and hypoxia. Even without adequate circulation, each cell may break down subcellular parts and recycle those into new proteins or energy as required to survive"[6].

---

6 Fung, Jason. "Autophagy – a Cure for Many Present-Day Diseases?" *Diet Doctor*, 19 Dec. 2017, www.dietdoctor.com/autophagy-cure-many-present-day-diseases.

Although understanding this process may require a bit of studying and learning some terms which are quite complicated, you need to know that autophagy can be viewed as a cellular housekeeper, because of its main functions:

- to eliminate defective proteins and organelles
- to prevent the accumulation of abnormal protein aggregates
- to eliminate intracellular pathogens

That sounds interesting, however, you are probably still asking yourself why you should force your body to do this process (as it has to be induced somehow). The list of benefits is very long, but you can see them all below:

- "Providing cells with molecular building blocks and energy
- Recycling damaged proteins, organelles, and aggregates
- Regulating functions of cells' mitochondria, which help produce energy but can be damaged by oxidative stress
- Clearing damaged endoplasmic reticulum and peroxisomes
- Protecting the nervous system and encouraging the growth of brain and nerve cells. Autophagy seems to improve cognitive function, brain structure, and neuroplasticity.

- Supporting the growth of heart cells and protecting against **heart disease**
- **Enhancing the immune system** by eliminating intracellular pathogens
- Defending against misfolded, toxic proteins that contribute to a number of amyloid diseases
- Protecting stability of DNA
- Preventing damage to healthy tissues and organs (known as necrosis)
- Potentially fighting cancer, neurodegenerative disease, or other illnesses"[7]

Now, this list sounds very convincing, especially since most of the benefits mentioned in it are backed up by research studies. You are probably wondering right now, how to induce autophagy and experience all its benefits. Specialists suggest that there are 3 ways to trigger the autophagy process.

"When does autophagy occur? Autophagy is active in all cells but is increased in response to stress or nutrient deprivation (fasting or starvation). This means you can utilize 'good stressors' like exercise and temporary calorie-restriction

---

7 Levy, Jillian. "Benefits of Autophagy, Plus How to Induce It." *Dr. Axe*, 4 Sept. 2018, draxe.com/benefits-of-autophagy/.

(fasting) to boost autophagic processes. Both of these strategies have been linked with benefits like weight control, longevity, and inhibition of many age-associated diseases."[8]

The first way to induce autophagy is through intermittent fasting. Restraining yourself from eating food for a while will eventually trigger autophagy. It's said that after 24 hours since your last meal, the autophagy process will start. This is probably the best way to induce autophagy, as it's a lifestyle habit that you completely control. Just like mentioned above, you will need to fast for a longer period in order to trigger autophagy. That's why it is recommended to use the Alternate Day Fast or Water Fasting in order to start autophagy. If you do choose the Alternate Day Fast, make sure you don't eat anything at all during the 36 hour fast, and make sure you don't consume any calories either. So try to stay away from juices or other soft drinks, as they are very high in sugar. If you do try the water fasting method, make sure you stick to it for at least 2 or 3 days, as the recommended fasting period, in this case, is 24 to 48 hours. For your own health and to induce autophagy, you should try the Alternate Day Fast, with no

---

8 Levy, Jillian. "Benefits of Autophagy, Plus How to Induce It." *Dr. Axe*, 4 Sept. 2018, draxe.com/benefits-of-autophagy/.

calories in the fasting window, or if you feel up to it, you can try the water fasting program for 2 to 3 days, once every 3 months. Just judging by the list of benefits this process has, I believe it's totally worth it to restrain yourself from eating for a period of 36, 48 or 72 hours.

The second way of triggering autophagy is the **ketogenic diet**. Although this type of diet will be detailed in a later chapter of this book, you still need to understand the basics of this meal plan (also known as the keto diet). The basic principle of this dietary plan is to cut down on carbs, therefore this diet suggests a low carb high fat intake. Basically, it suggests replacing the carbs with healthy fats, in order for the body to burn fat. How is this possible? Well, apparently once the body switches the primary fuel type from glucose to fat, it will just start to burn fat. It's up to you how much fat you consume in order for your body to burn more of your own fat reserves. The keto diet induces the metabolic state of ketosis, during which the ketone bodies are multiplying and the insulin level is decreasing. Once the insulin level gets low enough, the insulin will become active and will start to regulate (lower) the blood sugar level, and therefore decrease the risk of diabetes. Ketones are just some organic compounds produced by your liver capable of breaking down the fat tissue in order to release the energy stored therein. The keto-adaptation process is when your body runs on ketones and fats, whether we're talking dietary fat or fat tissue. Speaking of dietary fat, the keto diet requires 75% of your daily nutrient intake to be lipids, and just 5 to 10% to be carbs. The rest can be proteins. I know it sounds strange. How can you eat that much fat and still *burn* fat, and lose weight? The body simply won't notice the difference between your fat reserves and the ones you consume, so it will burn them nevertheless. Olive oil, coconut or almond oil should be something you consume a lot more often. Also, avocado, high-fat cheeses, nuts, seeds, and other types of vegetables should be consumed. More on the keto ingredients can be found in a later chapter of this book. "In response to such severe carb restriction, you'll begin to start producing ketone bodies that have many protective effects. Studies suggest that ketosis can also cause starvation-induced autophagy, which has neuroprotective functions. For example, in animal studies when rats are put on the ketogenic diet, the keto diet has been shown to start autophagic pathways that reduce brain injury during and after seizures."[9]

"Another 'good stress' that can induce autophagy is exercising. Recent research has shown that 'Exercise induces autophagy in multiple organs involved in metabolic regulation, such as muscle, liver, pancreas and adipose tissue. While exercise has

---

9 Levy, Jillian. "Benefits of Autophagy, Plus How to Induce It." *Dr. Axe*, 4 Sept. 2018, draxe.com/benefits-of-autophagy/.

many benefits, it's actually a form of stress because it breaks down tissues, causing them to be repaired and grow back stronger. It's not exactly clear yet how much exercise is needed to boost autophagy, but research does suggest that intense exercise is probably most beneficial. In skeletal and cardiac muscle tissue, as little as 30 minutes of exercise can be sufficient to induce autophagy.'"[10] Most people who try intermittent fasting are also able to work out, and once they get used to it, they will feel more energetic and will have the extra motivation to exercise and fast. If you combine all of them together, you should be able to induce autophagy even faster.

There are plenty of things to find out about autophagy, and you also need to know about its 3 main pathways:

1. " mTOR – sensitive to dietary protein
2. AMPK – 'reverse fuel gauge' of the cell
3. Insulin-sensitive to protein and carbohydrates

When these nutrient sensors detect low nutrient availability, they tell our cells to stop growing and start breaking down unnecessary parts – this is the self-cleansing pathway of autophagy. Here's the critical part. If we have *diseases of excessive growth*, then we can reduce growth signaling by

---

10 Levy, Jillian. "Benefits of Autophagy, Plus How to Induce It." *Dr. Axe*, 4 Sept. 2018, draxe.com/benefits-of-autophagy/.

activating these nutrient sensors. This list of diseases includes – obesity, type 2 diabetes, Alzheimer's disease, cancer, atherosclerosis (heart attacks and strokes), polycystic ovarian syndrome, polycystic kidney disease, and fatty liver disease, among others. All these diseases are amenable to *dietary intervention, not more drugs*".[11]

Analyzing each pathway of autophagy, you probably never heard of mTOR or AMPK, but I can bet that you are very aware of the term insulin. mTOR stands for the mechanistic or mammalian target of rapamycin and its definition it's pretty complicated to understand, as it involves nutrition and medical terms which you are probably not aware of. However, a common definition would sound like this: "A protein that helps control several cell functions, including cell division and survival, and binds to rapamycin and other drugs. mTOR may be more active in some types of cancer cells than it is in normal cells. Blocking mTOR may cause cancer cells to die. It is a type of serine/threonine protein kinase".[12]

------

11 Fung, Jason. "Autophagy – a Cure for Many Present-Day Diseases?" *Diet Doctor*, 19 Dec. 2017, www.dietdoctor.com/autophagy-cure-many-present-day-diseases.

12 "NCI Dictionary of Cancer Terms." *National Cancer Institute*, www.cancer.gov/publications/dictionaries/cancer-terms/def/mtor.

AMPK is another difficult term to understand, as it's something similar enough to mTOR. "AMP-activated protein kinase (AMPK) is an energy sensor that regulates cellular metabolism. When activated by a deficit in nutrient status, AMPK stimulates glucose uptake and lipid oxidation to produce energy, while turning off energy-consuming processes including glucose and lipid production to restore energy balance. AMPK controls whole-body glucose homeostasis by regulating metabolism in multiple peripheral tissues, such as skeletal muscle, liver, adipose tissues, and pancreatic β cells — key tissues in the pathogenesis of type 2 diabetes. By responding to diverse hormonal signals including leptin and adiponectin, AMPK serves as an intertissue signal integrator among peripheral tissues, as well as the hypothalamus, in the control of whole-body energy balance."[13]

If there are 3 pathways for the autophagy process, there are also several types of autophagy like microautophagy, macroautophagy, and chaperone-mediated autophagy.

---

13 Long, Yun Chau, and Juleen R Zierath. "AMP-Activated Protein Kinase Signaling in Metabolic Regulation." *The Journal of Clinical Investigation*, American Society for Clinical Investigation, 3 July 2006, www.ncbi.nlm.nih.gov/pmc/articles/PMC1483147/.

"Macroautophagy is 'an evolutionarily conserved catabolic process involving the formation of vesicles (autophagosomes) that engulf cellular macromolecules and organelles.' This is usually the type we hear the most about. Humans are not the only species to benefit from autophagy. In fact, autophagy has been observed in yeast, mold, plants, worms, flies, and mammals. Much of the research to date on autophagy has involved rats and yeast. At least 32 different autophagy-related genes (Atg) have been identified by genetic screening studies. Research continues to show that autophagic process is very important responses to starvation and stress across many species".[14]

As you probably know, insulin is a hormone responsible for allowing glucose in your blood to enter your cells and energize them to functioning properly. The more glucose you get, the more likely it is to get stored in your blood and to raise the blood sugar and insulin levels. Paradoxically speaking, higher levels of insulin will not mean a more active hormone. Only after its level *decreases* does insulin get active and starts to "work its magic," regulating the blood sugar level.

---

14 Levy, Jillian. "Benefits of Autophagy, Plus How to Induce It." *Dr. Axe*, 4 Sept. 2018, draxe.com/benefits-of-autophagy/.

These are the pathways of autophagy, but have you ever wondered what kind of foods you need to eat in order to induce autophagy? As you can imagine, all the food you need to eat has to be low carb. You can see below a list of foods and drinks which are known to induce autophagy:

- berries and other fruits: cherries, cranberries, elderberries, blackberries, strawberries, blueberries, and raspberries
- herbs and spices: rosemary, basil, coriander, cilantro, thyme, parsley, cardamom, cumin, turmeric, cinnamon, ginger, ginseng, black pepper, and cayenne pepper
- drinks: coffee and tea. Coffee needs to be without anything, so no sugar, milk or cream. The same rule applies to tea, but it's better to be herbal, black or green tea. Try to avoid fruit tea, as it's too sweet. You can also have apple cider and distilled vinegar
- alcoholic drinks: red and white wine, gin, vermouth, and vodka.

These are just a few food and drink types you can try for inducing the autophagy process, but you may also try to some other ones which are very healthy for your body. You can find them grouped below:

- veggies (tomato, squash, spinach, peas, pickles, bell pepper, green beans, beetroot, turnip, and carrots)
- fruits (avocado, olive, coconut, watermelon, honeydew, cantaloupe)
- nuts and seeds: almonds, Brazil nuts, cashews, chestnuts, chia seeds, flax seeds, hazelnuts, Macadamia nuts, peanuts, pecans, pine nuts, pistachios, pumpkin seeds, sesame seeds, sunflower seeds, walnuts
- almond butter, peanut butter, cashew butter, Macadamia nut butter
- milk and dairy: buttermilk, blue cheese, brie cheese, cheddar cheese, Colby cheese, cottage cheese, cream cheese, feta cheese, Monterey Jack cheese, Mozzarella, Parmesan, Swiss cheese, Mascarpone, cream, heavy cream, sour cream, whole milk, skimmed milk
- fats: butter, ghee, lard, beef tallow, avocado oil, cocoa butter, coconut oil, flaxseed oil, Macadamia oil, MCT oil, olive oil, red palm oil, coconut cream, coconut milk
- drinks: almond milk, almond water, coconut water, coconut milk, kombucha;
- protein shakes with water: whey protein shake, rice protein shake, hemp protein shake, pea protein shake, micro greens blend
- alcoholic drinks: beer, champagne, rum, cognac, tequila, chocolate liquor, mint liquor

Chapter 6 How to Start Intermittent Fasting?

You are probably not satisfied with the previous diets you had, as they were probably too radical, or they just didn't deliver the results you expected. Promising 10 or 20 pounds per week in weight loss is something very bold, which first of all, doesn't apply to all bodies. Therefore, having the right expectations is really important. Always keep in mind that most diets are to be followed on a short term basis, as they don't provide health benefits, but on the contrary, they can even do some damage to your overall health. On top of that, immediately after breaking the diet, you will start to gain weight again. So you lose weight only as long as you are on a diet.

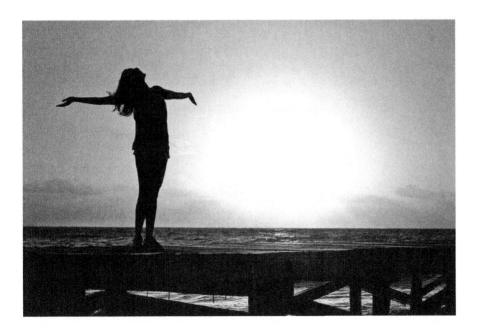

Processed food is abundant nowadays, and causes obesity on a large scale. A sedentary lifestyle combined with consuming so much processed food, and stress added, can lead to obesity. However, you don't have to be obese to start practicing intermittent fasting. One of the main principles of this way of eating is to focus on health, rather than the fat loss process itself. It's believed that a healthy body is more likely to function properly and even lose weight, so that's why IF is conducive to a healthy and sustainable weight loss. There are plenty of programs you can try when it comes to intermittent fasting, but you also need to know some important facts related to this practice:

- IF is more of a lifestyle, so it's way more than a diet
- it doesn't involve any meal requirements, as it's more about scheduling your meals, than what you eat
- don't expect miracles in terms of the weight loss process, as you will not have spectacular results. However, the fat burning process is more sustainable and a lot healthier than other diets
- it's highly recommendable to associate intermittent fasting with exercising;
- although there is no mention of any food requirements, it's highly recommendable eat healthy food, so trying a Mediterranean, keto or alkaline diet may be very good for this procedure

Such a procedure can be practiced by most people, depending on the program you choose to follow. However, some persons are not eligible for this practice:

- Pregnant women. Food deprivation is not something recommended for this category, as this is not the time to restrain themselves from food.
- Breastfeeding women. When they are breastfeeding, women really need all the possible nutrients they can get from food, so the babies get the best from breast milk.
- Women with an eating disorder like anorexia. When you are already underweight, you shouldn't be practicing intermittent fasting, as the process can lead you to even further weight loss, which may not be healthy.
- Underaged women. A growing body needs all the nutrients it can get from healthy food. Food deprivation is really not recommended in this case.

Depending on what exactly you are looking for, you can choose from any one of the intermittent fasting programs. If you prefer the daily fast, as you don't feel capable of fasting for a longer period, then perhaps the Leangains program is the right one for you. You have 8 hours to eat, and 16 hours of fasting. Daily fasts can be effective, especially if you associate it with an intense workout. Women can try cardio or endurance workouts, but swimming, jogging, Pilates and other types of physical activity are really recommended in this situation. If you feel that you can fast for more than 16 hours, then you can try the Warrior Diet, which is like an extension of the Leangains program. It limits the feeding window to just 4 hours, so you have 20 hours of the daily fast. If the previous program requires you to skip a meal, with the Warrior Diet you can only include 1 meal because you simply can't include any other main meal in just 4 hours. You can also add a snack, but still, the diet is too radical to be suitable for all women.

If you fancy fasting for a longer period, you can try the Alternate Day Fast, which includes 36 hours of fasting, or you can try the 24 hour fast. How frequent you want to have fasting days during your week is entirely up to you. For better results, you may need to add as many as possible. The Alternate Day Fast may induce autophagy, but to be sure you may need to try water fasting for 2-3 days once in a while. The second day of water fasting may be the hardest one, as you feel the most hunger. It's only up to your mind how you set it to overcome the situation and ignore the hunger. If you keep your mind occupied, you might get used to fasting, as you will not be tempted to eat and therefore, you will be able to keep on fasting. There are some side effects when it comes to fasting for a longer period, and you will experience fatigue, dizziness, and hunger. The secret to overcoming them is in your mind. If you are ambitious enough, if you are able to think of something other than the food, at some point you will get used to the fasting process, so you will no longer experience the situations mentioned above.

Intermittent fasting has plenty of benefits, but also a few side effects. You may need to try more programs to find out the one that best suits your needs. Trying a daily fasting program, associated with physical exercise and keto or Mediterranean diet can have better results in terms of fat loss, than trying a water fasting program for a long period. When you are on a water fasting program, if you do exercise, you won't have optimal performance, so your workout will not be very effective. A program which works wonders for another person, may not deliver the same results to you, or it will not have the results you expect. That's why you may need to try the several programs, before finding the one that fits your needs.

Probably the first one you will need to try is the 24 hour fast, but practiced just once a week. With intermittent fasting you will need to ease into it, so don't rush to try the hardest program, as you may not be up to it at first. After trying the 24 hour fast on a weekly basis (you can try it 3 or 4 weeks), you can switch to the Alternate Day Fast, but the mild version, as described by Dr. James B. Johnson, having just a few calories in the fasting days (or Down Days; it should be around 20% of the normal calorie consumption in the first weeks, then you can increase it to 35%). If you want to try fasting on a daily basis, you can try the Leangains program, which includes some meal scheduling for the feeding period. You will have 16 hours of daily fast, and if that's not enough, you can expand the fasting period to 20 hours per day, and transform your program into the Warrior Diet. You should try water fasting for a long period only as a last case scenario if you notice that these programs are not effective enough for you. However, you need the supervision of a physician to go on a water fasting for a longer period. Some people are able to fast for hundreds of days, consuming nothing but water and vitamins. Most doctors would not recommend water fasting for more than 72 hours, and if they consider that you need more than that, you definitely need their support and supervision in order to continue fasting for a longer period.

This is the recommended order to try the intermittent fasting programs in, but it's up to you how well you adapt to these programs. IF schedules the meals, but success also depends on what you eat, and if you work out. Combining all of these can have spectacular effects on your body, not only in terms of fat loss, but also in terms of overall health.

Chapter 7 Focus on Healthy Food

The human body needs macronutrients, minerals, and vitamins to function properly. All of them can be found in food, but unfortunately, the food available nowadays is not very consistent in nutrients. Most of the food we eat today is processed, and the more processed food is, the more unhealthy and less consistent in nutrients. Also, processed food is rich in carbs, a macronutrient which can cause terrible effects to the human body. In fact, food has killed more people over the last few decades than drugs, alcohol, and cigarettes put together. Around 70% of the diseases known today are caused by food.

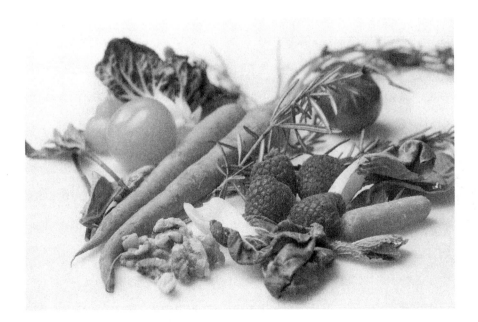

You are probably asking yourself why is this happening? The answer lies with processed foods and carbs, as they are the roots of all these problems. Carbs can be split into sugar and starch, and sugar really needs no introduction, as it's perhaps the most harmful substance ever to be consumed by humans. Without any doubt, food was a lot healthier 100 years ago, and there weren't so many cases of obesity and diabetes (both caused by an excess of carbs). The problem with sugar is that we consume it voluntarily and even feed it to our children. This kind of food causes addiction, as you will not feel satiety for a long time (in fact, you will feel hungry sooner), it won't cover the body's nutritional needs and you will crave some more carbs very soon. Those carbs contain glucose, which can be used by the body to generate energy, but this energy is produced only through physical exercise. The glucose doesn't get consumed and instead gets stored in your blood, raising your insulin and blood sugar levels. This is one step closer to diabetes, so this is how it all gets started.

Most of the food we consume today is processed and even what it claims to be natural is not organic. Before being able to process food, the most processed food you can dream of was bread, but the recipe was pretty simplistic, so different than the bread we are consuming today. Food was cooked from natural ingredients, and it had great nutritional value. Also, the lifestyle was a lot more active, as there weren't too many means of transportation back then. When we think of natural food nowadays, it's simply very difficult to find organic food, as chemicals are used to grow fruits, vegetables or crops. Fertilizers are no longer natural (with high chemical content), and animals are being fed concentrated food to grow incredibly fast. The meat we are consuming comes from these animals, and if they are fed this kind of food, this will affect us. Processing food is all about adding extra value to the product, otherwise, companies operating in this domain can't seem to find a way to increase their profits. It's fair to say that for the sake of profits, food processing companies are literally making poison to be consumed by the people. Everything which is packed and has more ingredients (many of them being chemicals you can't even pronounce) is processed food. This type of food is promoted by supermarkets and fast-food restaurants, as it fits perfectly with the current way of life. Finding healthy food is becoming a challenge nowadays, especially for the people who want to cut down on carbs. You are probably wondering what exactly you can eat in order to stay away from carbs.

Intermittent fasting is a procedure of self-discipline, in which you impose on yourself a strict set of rules and eat only within the designated feeding window. For most of the programs, there is no mention of what you can eat, however, this doesn't mean that you can stuff yourself with junk food. Healthy food can improve the results of this program, and there are a few options when it comes to healthy diets. You can consider a keto diet, a Mediterranean diet or an alkaline diet, and they all involve consuming plenty of vegetables and less meat. Most of them are LCHF (low carb high fat) diets, but the protein intake may vary from one diet to another. More details on the keto diet will be discussed in a future chapter of this book, but you can also consider utilizing a very well-balanced diet like the Mediterranean diet. This diet traces its roots from the living habits of the people living in the Mediterranean basin, so it doesn't mean just Italian cuisine. But be careful, as this diet doesn't include pizza and it doesn't focus on pasta. This kind of diet has its very own food pyramid, based on how frequent you should try that food type. If the standard food pyramid has 6 different levels like:

1) Vegetables, salad, and fruits
2) Bread, whole-grain cereals, pasta, potatoes, and rice - the food category richest in carbs
3) Milk, yogurt and cheese
4) Meat, poultry, fish, eggs, beans, and nuts
5) Oils, spread, and fats
6) Sweets, snacks, soft drinks, juices - basically food and drinks with very high levels of sugar and salt

The Mediterranean diet has it figured differently, as you can see below:

1) The base of the pyramid is represented by the physical activity, as this is a lifestyle for people living in the Mediterranean region.

2) The second level of the pyramid includes different types of food like fruits, vegetables, beans, nuts, olive oil, seeds and legumes, herbs and spices, but also grains (with a focus on whole grains). Most of the foods on this level should be consumed on a daily basis.

3) The third level of the pyramid is represented by seafood and fish, which should be consumed approximately twice a week.

4) The next level features poultry, cheese, yogurt, and eggs.

5) The last level of the pyramid is represented by meat and sweets.

The logic behind this pyramid is the same as with the standard food pyramid, the more necessary the food type is, the lower is on the pyramid. The Mediterranean diet includes a plethora of food types to choose from, all healthy, delicious and nutritious. Therefore, it's probably the most complete meal plan you can associate with intermittent fasting. You can eat fish, seafood, meat, chicken, turkey, but most of all, you will need to consume veggies, fruits, seeds, nuts, dairy products, and also olive oil. This diet focuses on healthy unsaturated fats, so it's exactly what the body needs for the IF lifestyle, as it can bring your body into ketosis (the metabolic state when ketones are multiplying to break down the fat tissue). Some of the main features of the Mediterranean diet are:

- focus on the consumption of fruits, nuts, veggies, legumes, and whole grains
- there is also a high emphasis on consuming healthy fats from canola or olive oil
- forget about the use of salt to flavor your food, as this diet encourages the use of herbs and spices
- less red meat (pork or beef) and more fish or chicken/turkey
- you can even drink red wine in moderate quantities

It doesn't sound like a diet at all, as there are so many types of food accepted. It's more of a lifestyle than a meal plan. If a standard diet is something you need to stick to for a few weeks, the Mediterranean diet is the meal plan that you have to stick to for the rest of your life. It can include all 3 meals of the day, but you can also have snacks or desserts. Sounds too good to be true? Well, this is what the Mediterranean diet is, and it can work wonders on you if you combine it with intermittent fasting and working out. But, that's not all! By now you already know the benefits of intermittent fasting. How about adding some more benefits by following this type of diet? If you want stronger bones, lower risk of frailty, lung disease or heart disease, and even to ward off depression, then you definitely need to try this diet.

Since this meal plan is very diversified, you don't have to make radical changes in your refrigerator, as you are probably already consuming some of the foods mentioned here. However, at least when it comes to veggies, legumes, and fruits, you will need to eat them fresh, so frequent shopping may be required. You need to know that the ingredients of the Mediterranean diet are structured into 11 categories, as you can see below:

1) **Vegetables** are one of the most important categories included in this meal plan and you can consume them frozen or fresh. In the frozen veggies group there can be included peas, green beans, spinach or others. In terms of fresh vegetables, you can buy tomatoes, cucumbers, peppers, onions, okra, green beans, zucchini, garlic, peas, cauliflower, mushrooms, broccoli, potatoes, peas, carrots, celery leaves, cabbage, spinach, beets, or romaine lettuce.

2) The **fruits** you need to include in your shopping list are peaches, pears, figs, apricots, apples, oranges, tangerines, lemons, cherries, and watermelon.

3) You can't have a Mediterranean diet without some high-fat **dairy** products. Milk (whether is whole or

semi-skimmed) is no longer considered a good option, as it also has a higher concentration of carbs. You can buy instead sheep's milk yogurt, Greek yogurt, feta cheese, ricotta (or other types of fresh cheese), mozzarella, graviera, and mizithra.

4) This diet doesn't focus too much on **meat or poultry,** but you can still eat them twice a week. Your shopping list will need to include chicken (whether you prefer it whole, breasts or thighs), pork, ground beef, and veal. This is where you can get most of your proteins from, but still, you need to keep the protein intake at a low level.

5) Can you imagine a Mediterranean diet without **fish or seafood**? Because this food type is a must in this meal plan, although you only have it twice a week. So, you will need to buy salmon, tuna, cod, sardines, anchovies, shrimp, octopus or calamari. You can eat some of them fresh or canned.

6) Although you don't have to abuse them, your shopping list should definitely include **bread or pasta**. If they are made from whole grains even better, as they are the right choice in this case. Try to avoid the unnecessary consumption of pastry, like having bagels, pretzels or croissants with your coffee. You can eat and buy instead whole grains bread, paximadi (barley rusks),

breadsticks (also made from whole grains), pita bread, phyllo, pasta, rice, egg pasta, bulgur, and couscous.

7) Your shopping list must include **healthy fats and nuts**. Olive oil should be consumed on a daily basis, so you need to have it in your household. Also, in terms of nuts, it's recommended that you buy tahini, almonds, walnuts, pine nuts, pistachios, and sesame seeds.

8) **Beans** are an important part of this diet, so you definitely need to buy lentils, white beans chickpeas, and fava.

9) **Pantry items** are the miscellaneous part of this meal plan. In this group, you can include olives, canned tomatoes, tomato paste, sun-dried tomatoes, capers, herbal tea, honey, balsamic or red wine vinegar and wine (preferably red).

10) As mentioned above, **herbs and spices** are used for flavoring your food. As this diet involves a lot of home cooking, having plenty of spices and herbs can make a difference. That's why your shopping list must include herbs and spices like oregano, mint, dill, parsley, cumin, basil, sea salt, black pepper, cinnamon, sea salt and all kind of spices.

11) You definitely need to buy some greens, like chicory, dandelion, beet greens and amaranth and include them in your meal plan.

Chapter 8: Calories

Any type of processed food is literally a calorie bomb, as the food is rich in calories, but it's very poor in terms of nutrients. Eating more calorie-dense foods will not keep the hunger away for a longer time, in fact, you will feel the hunger again faster than you think. When studying the label of any processed product, we can see the nutritional value table.

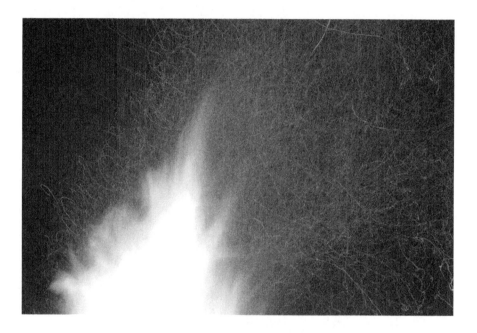

You will quickly notice that the food you are consuming is extremely rich in calories, but you will also notice really low values for proteins and sometimes even fats. Eating plenty of calories will not guarantee you extra energy, but burning them will. So why eat plenty of unnecessary calories per day, when you know that they are not going to be burned in full? You are probably wondering what is the normal calorie intake for the average woman. The answer depends on the muscle mass, height, and other factors. "An average woman needs to eat about 2000 calories per day to maintain, and 1500 calories to lose one pound of weight per week. An average man needs 2500 calories to maintain, and 2000 to lose one pound of weight per week. However, this depends on numerous factors. These include age, height, current weight, activity levels, metabolic health, and several others."[15]

Calories are units that measure energy and can be found in most food and drinks. People nowadays don't pay too much attention to how many calories they are consuming. Not only is processed food way too high in calories, but people may also snack often and drink soft drinks or juices, products which are also rich in calories. The lack of physical activity leaves too many calories unburned, and this is how the fat cells are accumulating.

---

15 Gunnars, Kris. "How Many Calories Should You Eat Per Day to Lose Weight?" *Healthline*, Healthline Media, 6 July 2018, www.healthline.com/nutrition/how-many-calories-per-day#section1.

Obesity is a major problem over the past few years, and unfortunately, it looks like it will continue to remain an even more serious problem in the years to come. The major problem with the food today is its quality, it is very calorie dense, not nutrient dense. It will not maintain the satiety level for a longer period, and it will make your body crave food again in short order. People often snack during such moments, and probably the most dangerous type of snack is a bag of chips. The calorie level skyrockets and more and more people have problems controlling their weight. The energy from the calories gets stored in your blood (in the form of blood sugar) or in the fat tissue, where you need special help from ketones to release the energy stored in there.

If you were used to eating plenty of calories per day, then you definitely need to lower the amount to approximately 2000 calories per day, or 1500 if you are planning to lose weight. Keeping the calorie intake at this level will either maintain your weight, or you can start to lose weight. Trying intermittent fasting doesn't mean that you need to eat more calories in the feeding period in order to compensate for the calorie intake for the lack of it in the fasting period. The eating window will need to be as on a normal day, the standard calorie intake, in order to make the IF program more efficient. Below you can find some of the best tips to control your calorie intake:

- focus on natural food, not processed. Following a special diet low in carbs can be the right thing, so an alkaline, Mediterranean or keto diet might be exactly what you need to keep the control of calories

- keep track of how many calories you are consuming. Although natural food is not packed as processed food is, you still need to browse for information over the internet to find out how many calories a steak or a salad may have

- rule out junk food. This type of food is the most calorie-dense food out there, and in terms of nutrients is very poor

- if you feel the need to snack, always use fruits, veggies, nuts, or smoothies. Forget about chips and other types of processed snacks

- make sure you avoid soft drinks or juices with high sugar levels. They are also very high in calories

It's hard to resist the temptation of consuming processed food since it's so popular and readily available. Completely eliminating pizza, burgers, donuts, chips, and soft drinks can be something very hard to do, as most of us really love all these kinds of foods, and we are addicted to them. Small things can make a difference, like not using sugar, milk or cream with your coffee, or eating natural meat, instead of processed ones (like sausages or meatballs). As a word of advice, don't even bother with reading the label of processed food. It will literally scare you because of the very high calorie level. Instead, shop around for fruits, veggies, and meat (although you don't have to eat too much of it). In many cases, when you have a steak, you shouldn't have French fries (or any type of cooked potatoes) or rice as a side dish, since these foods are rich in carbs and also high in calories. Instead have some grilled veggies (like peas, broccoli, carrots, and so on), and this should significantly lower the calorie intake of that meal. By the way, meat shouldn't be consumed on a daily basis, and even when you consume it, try to avoid frying it in oil (vegetable or sunflower oil). A keto diet should help you a lot with the calorie intake, but more details regarding this very popular diet can be found in the next chapter.

Chapter 9 Keto Diet

If you want to better understand why you need to follow a ketogenic diet, you need to first understand terms like ketosis and ketones. "Ketosis is a metabolic state in which your body uses fat and ketones rather than glucose (sugar) as its main fuel source. Glucose is stored in your liver and released as needed for energy.

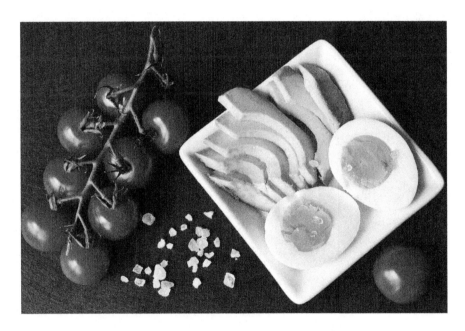

However, after carb intake has been extremely low for one to two days, these glucose stores become depleted. Your liver can make some glucose from amino acids in the protein you eat via a process known as gluconeogenesis, but not nearly enough to meet the needs of your brain, which requires a constant fuel supply. Fortunately, ketosis can provide you with an alternative source of energy".[16]

However, some specialists would disagree. They claim that ketosis is just the metabolic state with appropriate levels of insulin and ketones and the keto-adapted state is what makes the body run on fats.

Speaking of ketones, there are a few things you need to understand. "In ketosis, your body produces ketones at an accelerated rate. Ketones, or ketone bodies, are made by your liver from fat that you eat and your own body fat. The three ketone bodies are beta-hydroxybutyrate (BHB), acetoacetate, and acetone (although acetone is technically a breakdown product of acetoacetate). Even when on a higher-carb diet, your liver actually produces ketones on a regular basis – mainly overnight while you sleep – but usually only in tiny amounts. However, when glucose and insulin levels decrease on a carb-restricted diet, the liver ramps up its production of ketones in order to provide energy for your brain. Once the

---

16 Spritzler, Franziska, and Andreas Eenfeldt. "What Is Ketosis? Is It Safe? – Diet Doctor." *Diet Doctor*, 22 Mar. 2019, www.dietdoctor.com/low-carb/ketosis.

level of ketones in your blood reaches a certain threshold, you are considered to be in nutritional ketosis. According to leading ketogenic diet researchers Dr. Steve Phinney and Dr. Jeff Volek, the threshold for nutritional ketosis is a minimum of 0.5 mmol/L of BHB (the ketone body measured in the blood)".[17]

Now that we have this covered, the keto diet is one of the low carb high fat (LCHF) meal plans, and it is definitely one of the most popular diets nowadays. If done correctly, this dietary plan should provide you amazing results in terms of health management and weight loss. Just like intermittent fasting, the keto diet puts health first, as it's important for the body to achieve the right health status. You are probably wondering, what's the secret of this amazing diet? What exactly made it so famous? I will try to explain to you in this chapter, so you can easily understand its popularity.

The ketogenic diet is capable of reprogramming your body to run on fats instead of glucose, therefore it will burn body fat for energy, instead of glucose from carbs. The default fuel type of the body is glucose, especially with the food we eat today.

---

17 Spritzler, Franziska, and Andreas Eenfeldt. "What Is Ketosis? Is It Safe? – Diet Doctor." *Diet Doctor*, 22 Mar. 2019, www.dietdoctor.com/low-carb/ketosis.

You can find plenty of glucose in bread, pasta, potatoes, rice and all kinds of processed food. Unfortunately, almost everything we eat has a high or very high carb concentration. But, it's not just what we eat, it's also what we drink. Just think of all the juices and soft drinks with high sugar levels. So, glucose can come from carbs (when we consume too many of them), but it can also come from proteins. In other words, most of the food we eat today is very high in glucose. Energy comes from burning glucose, not from consuming it, so you will need to engage in physical activities in order to burn glucose, otherwise, it will get stored in your blood. This can lead to higher blood sugar, and this is where it all gets started when it comes to diabetes. Therefore, consuming high amounts of glucose is definitely not healthy for your body, so you need to find a way to replace it with a different energy source.

The ketogenic diet can provide you the alternative, as it's capable of replacing the carbs from your dietary plan with healthy fats. The ironic part is that you will lose weight. That's right! You will eat fat and lose weight! That's how the ketogenic diet works.

If you are wondering how this is possible, let me break it down for you. In the beginning of the chapter, there were some mentions about ketosis, the keto-adapted state and of course, ketones. Let's say that you radically change your diet, and you mostly eat fats. Since your body is so used to running on glucose, it will quickly notice that there is no more glucose to burn, since it's already stored in your blood, and that's not available to be consumed (insulin will take care of the glucose stored in your blood). Applying stress like controlled hunger (through intermittent fasting), or consuming dietary fat (using a keto diet), will activate the metabolic state of ketosis. The insulin level is decreasing until it eventually gets activated, while the ketone bodies are multiplying.

Now that you are consuming high levels of fat, your body will need to adapt to find a way to turn all this fat into energy. This is what the ketones are for. They are the only ones capable of breaking down fats and releasing the energy stored in there. Fats are easier to burn using the action of ketones than it was with glucose through physical activity. Switching the fuel type from carbs to fats is not easy. Although the modern Western diet is very poor in terms of nutrients (just rich in carbs) and you will not feel satiety for a long time, your body will crave more carbs once you feel hungry. At this point, it's addicted to carbs, so switching the fuel type to fats may not be something that it enjoys at first. There are plenty of reasons why you should cut down on carbs and replace them with fats. Once your body realizes that there is no more glucose to use, it will start burning fat for energy using ketones. If you don't eat anything, the ketones will act on your fat tissue, but if you eat keto food, it will burn through the dietary fat. Unlike glucose, which is no longer available once it gets stored in your blood, fats can be consumed and burned if they are already stored in your fat tissue, or if you just ate them. Once you have your body running on fats, keep feeding it mostly fats, and it will continue to run on this "fuel type." Just think of fats as the "biofuel" your body can use, as it will enhance your longevity, but it will also improve the function of your "engine" (which is the heart).

Speaking of benefits, you definitely need to check them below, just to have extra motivation to make this radical change to your diet.

The Benefits of the Ketogenic Diet

So far, we established the effects the keto diet has on your weight. You will start to lose weight once you switch to this diet. You can even try working out, to lose more weight and to accelerate the fat-burning process, but you also need to have the right expectations, as the keto diet is not a meal plan selling you false promises. Don't expect to lose 10 or 20 pounds per week. However, you will be able to notice some pleasant results once you climb on your scale.

It lowers the risk of prediabetes and diabetes

When dealing with such diseases and medical conditions, it's highly important to understand terms like insulin and high blood sugar. The modern Western diet "helps" you consume too much glucose, which will not get used (at least not all of it) and it will get stored in your blood. This is raising your blood sugar level until is too high above normal, which is a condition called high blood sugar, or in medical terms hyperglycemia. However, the body has the means to fight back (if you let it), so the pancreas can release insulin, which is a peptide hormone capable of lowering down the blood sugar level. Consuming too much glucose will also raise the insulin level, and the body becomes insulin resistant. In this phase, the insulin is not capable of fighting against the sugar (glucose) stored in your blood. Something has to change in order to reactivate the insulin.

Stopping the intake of glucose through intermittent fasting, or in this case, through the keto diet is exactly the kind of help insulin needs in order to get activated again, and to regulate the blood sugar level. In other words, glucose consumption is the cause, and the keto diet simply eliminates the cause and encourages the body to fight back using insulin. Although carbs may not be completely removed from your body, the glucose intake will be too low, and therefore it will be consumed immediately (and entirely), so you don't have to worry about getting more of it to your blood. The percentage of a keto meal plan should be at 75% fats, just 5 -10 % carbs, and the rest should be proteins. Obesity goes hand in hand with different medical conditions like diabetes, heart diseases, and many others. When you see the ads on social media, promoting all kind of diets promising you to lose 10-20 pounds per week guaranteed, what proof you have to support that?

As it turns out, all the benefits of the keto diet are backed up by science, so there were actual studies showing what results you can expect. There was a study conducted which concluded that people on a keto diet managed to lose 24.4 pounds, compared to 15.2 pounds lost by the people from the non-keto group (don't expect these results in a week, as the study was conducted for a period longer than a month). On top of that, 95% of the people on this diet were able to cut down on most of their diabetes medication, compared to just 62% of the people from the non-keto group. Another study also discovered a very interesting fact about the keto diet and diabetes: 7 people out of 21 renounced all diabetes medication after trying this diet.

The benefits of the keto diet don't apply just to weight loss and diabetes. There are plenty of other diseases or medical conditions which can be impacted by this dietary plan, as you can see below:

- Heart disease. Less body fat means a lower cholesterol level, but it can also lead to lower blood pressure and blood sugar. Therefore, the keto diet has a positive impact on blood circulation, and it can play an important role when it comes to preventing heart disease.

- Cancer. Remember, the keto diet can lead to autophagy and as mentioned in the prior chapter about this process, autophagy can prevent and even reverse cancer in an incipient phase. The ketogenic diet is capable of slowing down tumor growth, but also other types of cancer, assuming that they are in an incipient phase. There are plenty of cases when cancer is caused by the food we eat. Consuming healthy food is something highly recommended, and can help you prevent a terrible disease like cancer.

- Parkinson's and Alzheimer's diseases. Although it may sound a bit much, the keto diet is known to improve cognitive and mental function, therefore it can slow the progression of or even prevent neurodegenerative diseases like Alzheimer's and Parkinson's.

- Epilepsy. Several studies have shown the positive impact the keto diet has in reducing seizures for epileptic children, and also for adults.

- Polycystic ovarian syndrome can be caused by high insulin levels. Since the keto diet restricts carb consumption, this means that you will significantly lower the level of glucose. Lowering the glucose level will eventually lower the insulin level as well, and there will be a lower risk of polycystic ovarian syndrome.

- Brain injuries. Although the study was conducted on animals, the result is valid for humans too. There was a research that proved that the keto diet is able to decrease the effects of concussions and it can contribute to lower the recovery time after a brain injury.

- Acne. This condition may be caused by the excess of glucose in your blood. Since the keto diet is known for reducing the blood sugar and insulin levels, it can help with improving acne, and also other skin conditions. You can also induce autophagy by sticking to this diet, and this process has very impressive results on your skin, as it recycles and replaces the parts of the old cells, including at a skin level.

These benefits should determine everyone to radically change their meal plan and switch to the keto diet. However, you will probably need to make some serious changes in your refrigerator and your spices cabinet as your shopping list must include: almond butter, almond milk, almond butter, beef sticks (you must check the label for the carbs count), beef jerky, blackberries, cocoa nibs, cheese wedges, cheese slices, cheese chips, Brazil nuts, coconut oil, deli meat, dark chocolate, Greek yogurt, flaxseed crackers, cottage cheese, kale chips, Macadamia nuts, sugar-free Jell-O, olives, meat bars, Macadamia nut butter, peanut butter, pickles, pecans, pepperoni slices, protein bars (keep an eye on the carbs level), pork rinds, pumpkin seeds, seaweed snacks, sardines, smoked oysters, sunflower seeds, eggs, string cheese, walnuts, cauliflower, broccoli, avocado, mushrooms, toasted coconut flakes, string cheese, guacamole (pay extra attention to the carb levels), peppers and many other fruits or vegetables.

The fun part with the keto diet is that you can have all of the main meals, plus desserts and snacks. There are plenty of books providing plenty of keto recipes. You can follow them and prepare really delicious and nutritious food. Usually, people associate snacks with a very unhealthy habit of eating chips, sweets and drinking juices or soft drinks with very high sugar intake. The big problem with the modern-day diet is that the food is only calorie dense, not nutrient dense. It gives you the false impression of satiety, but that will not last for long. Carbs can cause addiction, and you will not feel satisfied, so you will need to eat more carbs. Even though it may be a challenge, there are snacks and desserts which are keto, so they are high in fats and low in carbs. Snacks and desserts can perpetuate the metabolic state of ketosis, as you will consume more fats. The keto diet can be a very important part of the "health triad", 3 elements that can help you become more healthy and lose more weight. The 3 elements of this health triad are intermittent fasting, the keto diet and physical exercise. All these combined can help your body enter ketosis, can help with the keto-adaptation process and eventually induce autophagy. Whether you want to combine this meal plan with IF and exercising, or you would like to stick just to the keto diet, you will experience plenty of benefits by trying this dietary plan.

Chapter 10 Muscle Gain

Intermittent fasting means food deprivation, and you need a daily intake to maintain your muscle mass. People mostly think that this procedure will cause muscle loss, not just fat burning. Well, they couldn't be more wrong! You are probably asking yourself, how is this even possible? Even though you are not eating the daily recommended intake of protein required to preserve your muscles, you will still not lose any muscle mass. Let me explain why.

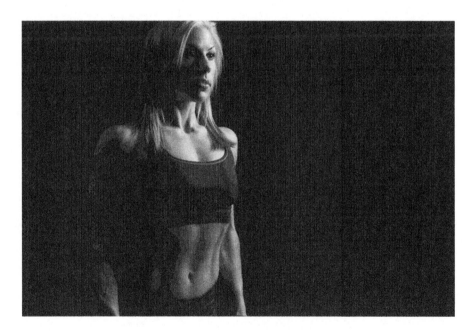

When people tell you that they want to lose weight, they want to lose *fat*. Most of the studies on this indicate that intermittent fasting programs are conducive for losing weight. However, the question you need to ask yourself is what kind of weight are you willing to lose? Losing muscle is not something that you can benefit from in most cases, so you are definitely wanting just to lose fat.

Physical exercise is highly important, as it can make the difference between losing muscles and fat, or losing just fat. Without exercise, you can lose the whole package through intermittent fasting, so you can experience both lean mass and fat mass loss. The lean mass includes the muscles as well. Working out can turn fats into muscles, so you can at least preserve or even expand your muscle mass through physical exercise. If you pair it with IF, then most likely your body will burn fat on a massive scale and will preserve your muscles. You will probably need to try high-intensity workouts in order to avoid muscle loss, but you will also need to remember that the growth hormone levels get very high through intermittent fasting. For example, after 48 hours of continuous fasting, the growth hormone level is 5 times higher than the one during the feeding window. This explains how your body will not lose weight if you work out intensely during the fasting period.

If you think about it, the prehistoric humans fasted a lot because they didn't have 3 main meals during the day, and it took a long time from one meal to another. They needed to hunt, fish or eat all sorts of foods, which were scarce and required some skills to acquire. The prehistoric human was a lot stronger than the modern-day human, even though they had to fast for longer periods. They had proper nutrient-dense food and had a very active lifestyle (which involved plenty of running, climbing trees or swimming). This is how intermittent fasting with exercise can be a very good combination to become stronger. Although there are better methods to gain weight, IF can prove to be a very effective way to pile on some muscle.

Several studies were conducted to find out how the human body reacts to food deprivation, so now we have some results of how the body reacts in a fasted state.

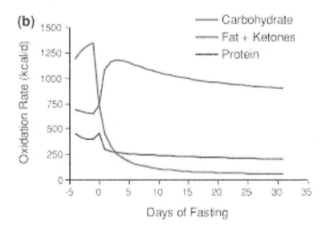

The graph above is taken from the "Comparative Physiology of Fasting, Starvation and Food Limitation" by Dr. Kevin Hall. It clearly shows where the energy is coming from in different moments of intermittent fasting. You can also notice that the body is using a mix of energy sources, mainly from carbs at the beginning, and then it uses the energy from fat and ketones.

"Within the first day or so of fasting, the body initially continues burning stored carbs for energy. Though, you'll notice that shortly after the body burns through those stored carbs it beings burning fat. This fat burning state is what drives diets like the Ketogenic diet. Meaning that in the absence of carbs your body has turned to a sort of 'backup generator' for energy, which is stored fat. So what about the protein (AKA muscle)? Well, while there is a low baseline of protein consumption there is no big spike in your body feasting on your muscle. In fact, this lowered baseline is an indicator of your body conserving muscle. Meaning that being in a fasted state doesn't automatically make your muscle wither away". [18]

Just like we mentioned above, gaining muscle mass through intermittent fasting may not be the best method, but it's still possible. You will need to set the right conditions and environment for your muscles to grow. This is why you need to make sure you have 3 factors in place: sufficient resources,

––––––––––––––––––

18 George, Lesley. "Intermittent Fasting And Muscle Gain: Go To Guide To Fasting Like A Pro • Shapezine - Digital Health & Fitness Tracking Blog." *Shapezine - Digital Health & Fitness Tracking Blog*, 10 July 2018, shapescale.com/blog/health/intermittent-fasting-muscle-gain/.

a positive nitrogen balance and the third one is to apply enough stress to the muscle mass in order to achieve hypertrophy.

The necessary resource for your body in terms of muscle growth is protein. Under normal circumstances, you will need to consume more proteins to gain more muscles. That's why bodybuilders stuff themselves with protein shakes or bars. However, during fasting, the situation is totally different. So it can get you confused and it will definitely make you wonder: "How can I be providing my body with enough food to grow muscle when I'm fasting? Well, providing your body with resources is more about the quantity of food rather than the timing. Meaning that you could fast for 8 hours in the morning then consume your caloric goal of 2,000 calories in the evening. Still maintaining that fasted state while also consuming enough calories to properly recover."[19]

When it comes to the positive nitrogen balance, it's all about eating more proteins than it is eliminating. So you need to make sure that you assimilate proteins and you are not

---

19 George, Lesley. "Intermittent Fasting And Muscle Gain: Go To Guide To Fasting Like A Pro • Shapezine - Digital Health & Fitness Tracking Blog." *Shapezine - Digital Health & Fitness Tracking Blog*, 10 July 2018, shapescale.com/blog/health/intermittent-fasting-muscle-gain/.

eliminating them through urine. This will eventually lead to muscle growth, so digesting proteins is what you need.

"Therefore, if we want to make sure we're in a positive nitrogen balance, we must simply consume enough protein. What this means for someone who is fasting is: consume enough calories during our 'feeding window' and pack in the protein. It's essentially the same as above. Just because you have a smaller window to consume protein doesn't mean you can't get enough. This way of eating simply concentrates your protein intake to a certain period. Instead of throughout the day."[20]

Have you ever wondered what the best way to gain muscles through training is? The answer is simple. You will need to use heavier weights, as applying more stress to the muscles will favor their growth. Make sure you add as much weight as you can lift, so try not to over-exaggerate, as you definitely want to avoid accidents or even hernias. Some specialists would agree that trying HIIT is the best way to grow your muscles through training. This involves having just a few repeats with very

---

20 George, Lesley. "Intermittent Fasting And Muscle Gain: Go To Guide To Fasting Like A Pro • Shapezine - Digital Health & Fitness Tracking Blog." *Shapezine - Digital Health & Fitness Tracking Blog*, 10 July 2018, shapescale.com/blog/health/intermittent-fasting-muscle-gain/.

heavy weights for about 20 seconds, then have 10 seconds break, then repeating the whole process again 8 times. So in 4 minutes, you can work a group of muscles very intensely. Others recommend progressive overload, which "means increasing the stress placed on the muscle through added weight. There are a number of ways that you can achieve progressive overload. However, the main two are: adding weight to the bar without sacrificing sets and reps or adding reps without sacrificing weight or sets. These are both great recipes to achieve efficient muscle growth. If you are achieving the above two factors of enough calories and protein, then there is no reason to have issues in progressing in your workouts. Even if you are actively practicing fasting."[21]

All of the conditions above set the right environment for your muscles to grow during intermittent fasting, whilst you are in the fasted state. Therefore, you will need to make sure that you will only get rid of the excess fat, not the muscle mass. You definitely need to work out very intensely, so if you want to gain muscles don't be afraid to deal with heavier weights.

---

21 George, Lesley. "Intermittent Fasting And Muscle Gain: Go To Guide To Fasting Like A Pro • Shapezine - Digital Health & Fitness Tracking Blog." *Shapezine - Digital Health & Fitness Tracking Blog*, 10 July 2018, shapescale.com/blog/health/intermittent-fasting-muscle-gain/.

Having too many repetitions with lighter weights will not do you any good in terms of muscle growth. You probably don't want to develop the body of a weightlifter, but you will still need to use heavier weights for better results in terms of muscle gain.

The next thing you will need to make sure you master is the energy dosage and a very important tip is to master the caloric cycling process, which basically means setting up the quantity and timing of the eating periods. The basic idea is to consume more calories when you train (after your exercise) and fewer calories when you don't. The best time to work out is during the fasted state, so you definitely need to avoid any kind of nutrient intake before your workout. "The key idea here being, adjust your calorie intake to help your body recover after hard workouts and don't be afraid pack in the protein. On days that you don't train you can back off on the calories. Especially, the carbs. How this translates to being incorporated into a fasting-centered diet is by simply making sure you are fitting the appropriate calories in your feeding window. Pretty simple."[22]

---

22 George, Lesley. "Intermittent Fasting And Muscle Gain: Go To Guide To Fasting Like A Pro • Shapezine - Digital Health & Fitness Tracking Blog." *Shapezine - Digital Health & Fitness Tracking Blog*, 10 July 2018, shapescale.com/blog/health/intermittent-fasting-muscle-gain/.

It's up to you to decide which intermittent fasting program works best for you in terms of muscle growth if you associate it with physical exercise. Probably the best programs are the daily fasting ones since they can provide you will all key requirements for your muscles to grow through IF. That's why the Leangains program and the Warrior Diet may be the right ones for you. Bodybuilders are huge fans of the Leangains program (also known as the 16/8 hour fast). It basically splits the day into an 8-hour feeding window and a 16-hour fasting period. This program may be the perfect example of caloric cycling, as it very clearly sets your feeding period and fasting period, but you can also plan to eat the most consistent meal of the day after your workout. If you want to burn fat and gain muscles at the same time, you can adapt your very own Leangains method:

- 8:00 - 9:15 am it can be workout time. You can train at your local gym, but don't be afraid to "play" with heavier weights.

- 10 am - the most consistent meal of the day. Forget about the typical breakfast, as you shouldn't eat cereals for breakfast. A protein boost is what you need, so a very consistent omelet with bacon and cheese seems to be the right choice.

- 2 pm - it's time for lunch. Grilled meat like chicken or pork, served with vegetables on the side can be the right choice. Don't forget about salad as an option.

- 6 pm - a light dinner. Take it easy with the calorie intake for this meal. When it comes to the meals of the day, make sure they are low on carbs, and higher on proteins and fats.

Your body should still run on fats, that's why the carb level should be at a minimum level. However, you will need to make sure that your protein intake gets assimilated by your body, and your muscles will begin to grow. Repeating the schedule above, working hard at the gym and also having the proper protein intake should definitely lead to muscle gain. To maximize your protein intake, you can also have a protein shake or bar between the meals. This is how you can make sure your muscles will grow through intermittent fasting.

Strangely enough, studies have shown that the growth hormone reaches unbelievably high levels if you fast for at least 48 hours. At that point, it's 5 times higher than it was in the feeding period. That sounds too good to be true, but most humans can't benefit from this situation, as they don't have the necessary resources at that point to engage in very intense training. If the growth hormone has very high levels, it may still not be enough to grow your muscles, as you will need intense training to take advantage of the high values of this growth hormone.

Chapter 11 Common Mistakes

Intermittent fasting is starting to become a very popular practice, however, it's important that it be understood and applied properly in order to take advantage of all its benefits, whether we're talking about weight loss, better digestion, fewer cravings, or lower inflammation. Truth be told, you should set your fasting window for as long as *you* feel comfortable with. Using a daily fasting program might be the easiest program to stick to, as you have just 16 hours of fasting period per day, which sounds totally doable.

Other programs involve increasing the fasting window to 20, 24 or 36 hours. Only the first one can involve daily fasting, as the other ones may involve fasting for once or twice a week if you feel up to simply quitting food for a longer period of time. It's true that the Alternate Day Fast (with a fasting window of 36 hours) may allow you to consume a minimum amount of calories in the fasting period (limited to just 500 calories in that day). Other people may want to consider the "purest" IF program, which is water fasting, but only a few people are capable of sticking to this one.

Whether you prefer daily fasting or longer term fasting, should be up to you. You may need to try a few intermittent fasting programs to find out which program best suits your needs. Also, you need to set the right expectations, as this program simply can't make false promises, so you can't expect to lose 10 or 20 pounds per week. It may not be the quickest weight loss program, but you can easily consider it one of the healthiest.

It's said that humans best learn from mistakes, so you can find below a list of the most common mistakes when it comes to IF:

1) Quitting too soon. Let's face it! Intermittent fasting is simply not easy, mostly because your body will need to run on just a few calories, or without any food at all for a longer-than-usual period. It's more about self-discipline, as you need to train your body and mind to overcome the stress of food deprivation, even if you feel

hungry. Once you practice this for more than a week (you can try daily fasting, not necessarily water fasting for more than a week), you will get used to it, and you will not feel as hungry and irritated anymore. If you are not reaching this phase, you probably chose the wrong IF program, and you may need to try a different one. Still, don't get discouraged, as there are high chances that one of the intermittent fasting programs might suit your needs.

2) Over-eating at meal time. This procedure will definitely make you experience hunger, but this doesn't mean that you need to stuff yourself with too much food, just because you are very hungry. Try not to compensate for the time you are not consuming calories, as you will rule out most of the benefits of intermittent fasting, especially the one related to weight loss. Dr. Brigitte Zeitlin is one of the specialists in this field of expertise, and she believes in the healthy principle of "fewer calories in than calories out." In other words, you will need to lower your calorie intake, as if you consume the same amount of calories or even more, you will definitely not lose weight at all. This procedure should lower the amount of food you consume during the day, and this means fewer calories. "Instead of piling food onto your plate when it's finally time to eat, portion out your meals so you know exactly what you're taking in

and avoid that whole 'eyes bigger than your stomach' situation. If you need a little help understanding how many calories to strive for—and what macronutrients those calories should consist of—Zeitlin suggests keeping a food journal or using an app like MyFitnessPal or Fitbit to get a clear picture of how your current food intake matches up to your goals and what nutrients you may need more or less of. And when you do sit down for your meals, take your time eating so your hunger cues have ample time to kick in and let you know if you truly need more."[23]

3) Eating insufficient amounts of food. The body still needs macronutrients, minerals, and vitamins from food in order to function properly. Intermittent fasting means food deprivation, but you don't need to overdo it. You still need to eat properly, even though you are trying any of the IF programs. This procedure is simply not for everyone, and most specialists don't recommend fasting for more than 72 hours. If someone

---

23 Lefave, Samantha. "8 Major Mistakes People Make When Intermittent Fasting." *What's Good by V*, 31 Jan. 2019, whatsgood.vitaminshoppe.com/intermittent-fasting-mistakes/.

is determined to fast for a longer period, this should only be done with the strict supervision of a physician. People should not try to radicalize this program, so they shouldn't eat too little. "'Some people don't want to undo what they've just done while fasting for hours or they have the mentality that if they eat too much the next fasting period will be harder," says Zeitlin. But consistently eating far below your calorie needs is a mistake, and kicks your body into 'starvation mode,' slowing your metabolism and making it that much harder to shed fat. Even if you're restricting when you eat your food, 'your body still needs an ample amount of food so your organs can function, and you can think straight and be the fantastic human that you are,' she says."[24] Not eating enough calories will cause you to feel irritable, weak and unable to focus.

4) Not consuming the right food. It goes without saying that some types of food should definitely be avoided. I'm referring of course to processed and junk food. Any type of packed food, with too many ingredients (some of them are impossible to pronounce) should be

---

24 Lefave, Samantha. "8 Major Mistakes People Make When Intermittent Fasting." *What's Good by V*, 31 Jan. 2019, whatsgood.vitaminshoppe.com/intermittent-fasting-mistakes/.

avoided, as they are incredibly high in carbs. However, food types like bread, pastry, pasta, potatoes, and rice should be consumed only moderately, as they also have high carb levels. Unfortunately, processed food is calorie dense and definitely not nutrient dense. This means they have too many calories compared to their nutritional value. These kinds of food will not make you feel satiety for a long time. In plenty of cases, you will feel the urge to snack soon after your last meal, and then react by consuming a bag of chips or eating some kind of sweets. Having a soft drink or a very sweet juice is probably the worst drink you can have with these snacks. It's a vicious circle because it encourages you to consume more carbs, more processed food and drinks, which will eventually affect your health. "Focus on eating a healthy balance of all the macronutrients (healthy fats, lean protein, and carbs) and fiber (which will help with satiety, gas, and bloating) your body needs to function well. Zeitlin suggests loading half your plate with veggies, a quarter with lean protein (think fish, chicken, and turkey), and a quarter with healthy starches like brown rice, quinoa, and sweet potato. If you're going to end up eating slightly fewer calories than usual, you need those calories to be as nutritious and body-serving as possible. Just because you're eating fewer calories doesn't mean those calories can come from sub-par sources."[25]

5) Not drinking enough fluids. Hydration is very important during intermittent fasting, and many beginners are thinking that they simply can't consume anything during fasting hours. Well, that's wrong! You don't have to fast strictly, leaving out water as well. In fact, there's nothing wrong with consuming water, coffee or tea during this period. However, there is a rule. Don't use any sugar, or any milk, cream or butter. In other words, don't add anything to your tea or coffee. Hydrating yourself can be a very useful tool when it comes to extending your feeling of satiety. Therefore, drinking water can help you get rid of the hunger feeling.

6) Going for the hardest program. Many people feel like they want to challenge themselves when taking on an intermittent fasting program, so they're fasting for several days during the week (I'm not referring to daily fasting, it's about fasting for at least 24 hours). The Eat-Stop-Eat program involves fasting for 24 hours twice a

---

25 Lefave, Samantha. "8 Major Mistakes People Make When Intermittent Fasting." *What's Good by V*, 31 Jan. 2019, whatsgood.vitaminshoppe.com/intermittent-fasting-mistakes/.

week, so it's fair to also call it the 5:2 program. Turning this program into 4:3, may not be something recommendable, in fact, it can even be dangerous. "'You're not supposed to starve yourself,' says Zeitlin. 'Our bodies require fuel to think straight, work well, converse normally, and move around—and that fuel comes from calories,' she says. Restricting your food intake too much takes a toll on your everyday life—and that's not what fasting is all about."[26]

7) Forcing the intermittent fasting programs. You need to understand right from the beginning that this procedure may not be the best when it comes to longevity, weight loss or metabolic health. It's a very sustainable method, but it doesn't work for everyone. Setting the right expectations is very important, as you know exactly what can be achieved through IF. That's why if you are trying an intermittent fasting program and you feel it's not delivering the results you expect, you need to stop trying this program and try another one. Starving yourself on a regular basis may not be the best way to get the benefits of this lifestyle. If you think

---

26 Lefave, Samantha. "8 Major Mistakes People Make When Intermittent Fasting." *What's Good by V*, 31 Jan. 2019, whatsgood.vitaminshoppe.com/intermittent-fasting-mistakes/.

of the prehistoric humans, they didn't have food on a regular basis, so they fasted involuntarily. For example, intermittent fasting may not be for people with strong appetites because they are not used to restraining themselves from food for a longer period of time.

8) Not switching to an active lifestyle. Plenty of diets can promise you will lose many pounds, as the food type they are promoting just burns fat without any effort. This isn't quite true. You may be able to eat food which is rich in fats, but without physical activity, it's all in vain. This is the right type of stress that can make your body burn fat. Even when you do exercise, the results are not very spectacular, as most people were able to lose just one pound per week.

9) You are not busy enough. This doesn't necessarily mean training, it can mean something else. During fasting, you might be tempted to think of food and it's very hard to resist the temptation of eating something. That's why you definitely need to stay away from the kitchen, or from any refrigerator or plate with food during the fasting period. Keeping your mind and body busy is what can get you through this procedure easily.

10) You abuse caffeine. If you have a very stressful lifestyle and you have your job to thank for this, then probably consuming coffee all the time is something very common for you. You have to get rid of this habit during

intermittent fasting, as you will need to stick to just 2 cups of coffee per day, with no sugar or anything else added. It goes without saying that you don't have to drink energy drinks, they have too many calories and are literally poison for your body. One of the purposes of intermittent fasting is to generate energy by burning fats, whether it's the fat tissue or dietary fat. The body is perfectly capable of producing its own energy, so you don't have to drink too much coffee, black tea, energy drinks, or any other kind of drink high in caffeine.

11) You are afraid of experiencing hunger. If you are asking yourself, why I should experience hunger, then this is not the right attitude for IF. "Hunger is a totally normal and natural part of life. Your muscles won't waste away. You will not die from fasting for 16-20 hours. Your body can survive extreme conditions. Some studies even show that going through stints without food can benefit health. *Short term* deprivation doesn't cause the body to break down muscle and go into 'freak out' mode and gobble up muscle tissue."[27]

---

27 Michal, Anthony. "9 Common Intermittent Fasting Mistakes." 26 Oct. 2017, anthonymychal.com/intermittent-fasting-mistakes/.

Chapter 12: Mindset and Tips

I think we can all agree that intermittent fasting is not an easy lifestyle to adapt to, and is definitely not for everyone, even though some are physically fit and healthy enough to try it. Everyone who tries to follow an IF program should be very determined and ambitious. You need to have the right attitude in order to make this procedure work for you. As you already know, mindset is a collection of thoughts and opinions which are reflected in your attitude.

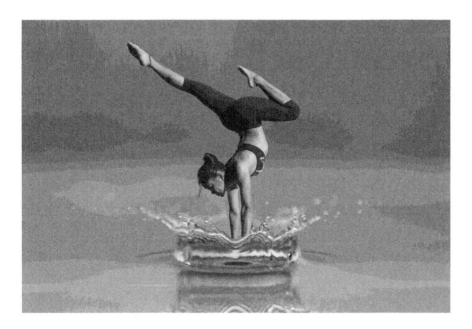

The power of will can get you through this process, regardless of the hardship you experience during IF. After all, intermittent fasting is more of self-discipline and a lifestyle, so it's not something you should only stick to it for a few weeks.

There is science behind this procedure, so it's not magic or "voodoo." Every benefit of it can be backed up by science, so if you follow the rules of it, you will most likely experience most of the benefits yourself.

The modern diet includes too much processed food. There are several issues with this type of food. It's unhealthy, it's very calorie dense (so it's high in calories), has little to no nutritional value and it will only keep the hunger away for a very limited amount of time. It causes addiction, as you will need to eat more (and repeatedly), in order to feel satisfied again, but while you are trying to achieve satiety, you are stuffing yourself with carbs (which contain a high amount of glucose).

The main purpose of fasting is to get your body in the fasted state. That's when the magic is happening, so that's when the fat burning process starts. The fasted state can only start 12 hours after your last meal, and this can be very challenging, especially if you are a person who likes to eat a lot and can't go without food for that long. This is when your brain comes into play, as this is the organ capable of not only ignoring or controlling the hunger feelings, but also your actions. So the brain will need to impose the food restrictions for the fasting period. There are several tips to help you go more easily through the intermittent fasting process. Below you can find a list of the most useful tips for achieving this:

1) Stick to shorter fasting periods. As there are several programs to fast, you should first try the ones with a shorter fasting window. This is how you can get used to fasting. You can try daily fasting, or fasting just once or twice per week. You can choose to fast for 16 hours (for the daily Leangains program) or 24 hours (for the Eat-Stop-Eat program or the 5:2 method, i.e., 5 days of normal feeding associated with 2 days of fasting). Trying to fast for more than 24 hours, like 48, 72 and even more hours, is not something that can be done by everyone. "Longer fast periods increase your risk of problems associated with fasting. This includes dehydration, irritability, mood changes, fainting, hunger, a lack of energy and being unable to focus. The best way to avoid these side effects is to stick to shorter fasting periods of up to 24 hours — especially when you're just starting out. If you want to increase your fasting period to more than 72 hours, you should seek medical supervision."[28]

---

28 West, Helen. "How to Fast Safely: 10 Helpful Tips." *Healthline*, Healthline Media, 2 Jan. 2019, www.healthline.com/nutrition/how-to-fast#section1.

2) Eat small amounts of food on your fast days. If you are on a daily fasting program, you will need to avoid any calorie consumption during the fasting window, but you will also need to lower the calorie intake for the feeding window. That's why you need to eat nutrient-dense food, so as natural as you can. Most processed food is very low on nutrients and high on calories, so the more natural you eat, the more nutritional value you will get. If you are using the Alternate Day Fast program, this one allows you to consume around 20% of your daily calorie consumption, from a normal feeding day. This method will lower the chances of hunger, dizziness and fatigue, side effects which are usually associated with intermittent fasting.

3) Proper hydration is a must. During intermittent fasting you should only consume water, tea or coffee (without anything added). If you don't hydrate yourself properly, you can experience headaches, dry mouth and also fatigue. The normal fluid intake is around 2 liters per day. However, around 20-30% of the necessary fluids come from your food, but it's not a mandatory rule. You can drink as much as your body demands. "As you meet some of your daily fluid needs through food, you can get dehydrated while fasting. To prevent this, listen to your

body and drink when thirsty."[29] Water can also be used to alleviate the feeling of hunger.

4) Meditation and walks can help with IF. When you are feeling hungry or bored, taking long walks or meditating can do the trick and help you get through the fasting period more smoothly. You definitely don't want to think of food, so you need to keep your mind busy through meditation, or you need to stay away from any source of food. Reading a book, listening to music or taking a bath can also help. This is how you can fast for days.

5) Don't feast if you plan to break the fast. There couldn't be a worse way to end the intermittent fasting program than breaking it with a huge meal. After a period during which you trained your body to run on a small number of calories, your stomach and digestive system are no longer used to processing a larger amount of food. So, if you want to feel tired and bloated, then go ahead and eat a copious amount of food. Naturally, a calorie bomb will prevent you from achieving any weight loss goals.

---

29 West, Helen. "How to Fast Safely: 10 Helpful Tips." *Healthline*, Healthline Media, 2 Jan. 2019, www.healthline.com/nutrition/how-to-fast#section1.

One of the main ideas behind IF is the calorie deficit: during this program, you will burn more calories than you consume. Breaking a fast should be just like when one starts the program, you will need to ease into it. Therefore, if you want to break the fast you will need to progressively increase your calorie intake until you are at the optimum level, or what is considered a normal level of calorie consumption. If you do want to quit practicing intermittent fasting, that's your call, but I would highly recommend continuing exercising at the very least.

6) Stop fasting if you are not feeling well. One of the main goals of IF is to make you feel better, but there are some side effects to it, like hunger, dizziness or headaches. If you fast for a longer period, you shouldn't keep on fasting regardless of how you feel. Therefore, if you are experiencing any of the symptoms above in an intense manner, you will need to stop immediately. You may experience these side effects if you fast for a longer period, like more than 24 hours. To limit such disadvantages, you might want to limit your fasting period to 24 hours. Remember, intermittent fasting is not for everyone, especially the ones with longer fasting periods. Even the Alternate Day Fast, which includes a fasting window of 36 hours, suggests some calorie intake during fasting. If you start to feel ill or faint, it's

always handy to keep a snack at hand. If intermittent fasting makes you feel ill, and you are starting to feel concerned regarding your health, then you need to stop fasting immediately. "Some signs that you should stop your fast and seek medical help include tiredness or weakness that prevents you from carrying out daily tasks, as well as unexpected feelings of sickness and discomfort."[30]

7) Make sure you consume enough protein. When people think of losing weight, they are thinking of burning fat, so they are referring to fat loss. Almost nobody wants to lose muscle mass. There are a few tricks to keeping or even growing muscle mass during IF, and one of them is consuming enough proteins. It's said that the body requires a certain amount of proteins to maintain its muscle mass. Intermittent fasting is a procedure of calorie deficit, which can lead to muscle loss, in addition to fat loss. Fasting days will definitely not have too many proteins, but there are some programs like the Alternate Day Fast which allow you to have a small calorie intake. You can associate that snack with a

---

30 West, Helen. "How to Fast Safely: 10 Helpful Tips." *Healthline*, Healthline Media, 2 Jan. 2019, www.healthline.com/nutrition/how-to-fast#section1.

protein shake or bar, just to make sure your body has enough proteins to preserve its muscle mass. Consuming food supplements like protein bars or shakes can be an excellent method to use to manage hunger. There are some studies which show that consuming approximately 30% of your meal's calories from protein can lead to a decrease in your appetite.

8) You will need to eat plenty of whole foods during non-fasting days. "Most people who fast are trying to improve their health. Even though fasting involves abstaining from food, it's still important to maintain a healthy lifestyle on days when you are not fasting. Healthy diets based on whole foods are linked to a wide range of health benefits, including a reduced risk of cancer, heart disease, and other chronic illnesses. You can make sure your diet remains healthy by choosing whole foods like meat, fish, eggs, vegetables, fruits, and legumes when you eat."[31]

9) You may need to consume supplements. Food restriction also means nutrient deprivation, so you will not get all the nutrients from your food such as

---

31 West, Helen. "How to Fast Safely: 10 Helpful Tips." *Healthline*, Healthline Media, 2 Jan. 2019, www.healthline.com/nutrition/how-to-fast#section1.

minerals, vitamins and of course the required macronutrients like proteins and healthy fats. Also, consuming fewer calories during the feeding window will definitely not cover your nutritional needs. Protein bars or shakes may not be the only supplements you will need to take, as your body could lack iron, calcium, and vitamins like B12. This is why is important to take multivitamin supplements, to make sure your body will not lack any mineral or vitamin. The best way to assimilate them is from your own food, by having a very well-balanced diet (The Mediterranean diet may be the ideal meal plan in this case because of the wide variety of foods it allows for).

10) If you are new to intermittent fasting, make sure you keep your exercises mild, not intense. Once you get used to IF you can try the intensive training to achieve very good results, but if you are new to this way of eating, just take it slow when it comes to exercising. As your body goes through important changes and it's experiencing nutrient deprivation, you may not have the required resources at the moment to train at maximum capacity. You can imagine that people who are water fasting will not be able to exercise properly on their 5th day of fasting. That's why newbies should try low-intensity (at the beginning) exercises, and add more intensity to your training as soon as you get used

to intermittent fasting. Walking, yoga and some stretching may be more than enough in the incipient phase. However, probably the most important tip related to working out is to always listen to your body and allow it to rest if it's feeling tired and struggling with exercises during the fasting window. It's highly recommended to work out during your fasting periods, but if you are new to fasting, keep it mild and gentle when it comes to these workouts during this period. When you get used to the IF lifestyle, you can slowly add some more intensity to your training.

11) Try a LCHF (low carb high fat) diet. When you are trying out the intermittent fasting programs, what you eat during the feeding window is important. Remember, the outcome of IF is to train your body to run on fats, so why not make it easier for it to do so? Ketosis is the metabolic state that encourages ketones to be active and break down the fats. These fats can come from your body's fat tissue or from the fat you eat. The activity of ketones over fats will generate energy. Speaking of dietary fat, you can get them with a proper LCHF diet like the keto diet (which is probably the most popular diet nowadays), or the Mediterranean diet. The keto diet replaces the carbs from your standard diet with fats, so you will have a nutrient ratio of approximately 75% fats and 5 - 10% carbs (the rest are

proteins). The Mediterranean diet is similar enough to the keto diet, but it doesn't have so much fat, and does allow a few more carb-rich foods. However, the carb level is still low enough for the body to achieve ketosis.

If you follow these tips you will most likely succeed in achieving the best results possible through intermittent fasting. However, as a bonus, here are some extra pieces of advice related to this lifestyle:

1) You will need to decide if it suits you. As you already know, intermittent fasting is not for everyone. Eliminating the people who are not physically fit or healthy enough to follow this lifestyle, it's also up to you to decide if you are eligible for any program of IF. Depending on your lifestyle, types of exercises you prefer and nutritional experience, you should be able to establish if this is for you. Find out the basics first, ask for information from a specialist, then decide if you want to go ahead with it.

2) Ease into it. If you are a newbie, you just heard of intermittent fasting and you are curious enough to try it, you need to start with the easiest possible program for you. You can try the daily fast of the Leangains program, or you can fast for only twice a week with the Eat-Stop-Eat program. See if scheduling your meals could be working wonders for you.

3) Concentrate on what every IF program has to offer, and don't get lost in details. All the intermittent fasting programs can eventually have the same benefits, but not all bodies respond in the same way to these programs. Considering that they all have the same benefits, you may need to try more than one program, until you find the right fit for you.

4) Remember to stay flexible. Flexibility, in this case, means to be able to easily switch from one program to another if you don't find a particular one delivering the results you expected.

5) Know yourself. Intermittent fasting is also about self-discovery, not just self-discipline. You can find out what your body's limits are and how it reacts in different situations (find out how long it takes to feel hunger, but also how it can overcome this situation).

6) Allow it some time to work. This is not a "super" diet promising you to lose 10-20 pounds per week. It takes time for its effects to take place, as this lifestyle mostly prepares your body for the fat-loss process. It's believed that a healthy body can perform better, so it puts health first then fat loss. Most people on intermittent fasting have only lost 1 pound per week, which is very slow from some people's point of view. This procedure is one of the most healthy and sustainable methods in terms of fat loss, but in order to fully experience all the health benefits as well, you will need to let it work and try it for a longer period of time.

7) You may experience ups and downs. Not everything with this procedure is "milk and honey." There are some ups and downs with it, just like everything else in life. Keep an open mind and don't freak out when you experience the downs. This is the only way you can focus on achieving the ups.

8) Set the right expectations, so think what exactly you want to achieve from doing this procedure. Intermittent fasting can be considered a very good way to:
   - "go deeper into the psychological and physical experience of true hunger
   - learn the difference between 'head hunger' and 'body hunger'
   - learn not to fear hunger
   - improve insulin sensitivity and re-calibrate your body's use of stored fuel
   - respect the process and privilege of eating
   - learn more about your own body;
   - lose fat, *if* you are careful about it
   - take a break from the work of food prep and the obligation to eat."[32].

---

32 Berardi, John, et al. "All About Intermittent Fasting, Chapter 11." *Precision Nutrition*, www.precisionnutrition.com/intermittent-fasting/appendix-b-tips-and-tricks.

9) "Respect your body cues. Pay attention to what your body tells you. This includes:

1. drastic changes in appetite, hunger, and satiety – including food cravings
2. sleep quality
3. energy levels and athletic performance
4. mood and mental/emotional health
5. immunity
6. blood profile
7. hormonal health
8. how you look"[33]

---

33 Berardi, John, et al. "All About Intermittent Fasting, Chapter 11." *Precision Nutrition,* www.precisionnutrition.com/intermittent-fasting/appendix-b-tips-and-tricks.

Conclusion

Is it really surprising for anyone out there why people nowadays are feeling so sick and are so vulnerable to diseases? Why we are experiencing these major issues when everything should be all about hygiene when it comes to food? How come people who lived 100 years ago didn't experience these issues we are experiencing today? These are all questions we should ask ourselves. The answer lies with the food we consume today.

As most of the food we consume today is processed, and it's far from being in a natural state, we can only think that this food is having harmful effects on our bodies. By harmful effects I mean obesity, heart, lung, liver, kidney and stomach diseases, diabetes, Alzheimer's and Parkinson's disease, and also different types of cancer. More than 70% of the diseases we know today are caused by processed food and high carbs concentration. In fact, processed food has killed more people than cigarettes, drugs, and alcohol put together.

What we think is natural food is not natural at all, so it has been replaced with the term "organic food." Let's think about it, as agriculture uses chemical fertilizers and pesticides on fruits, vegetables, and crops. Animals are being with concentrated food to grow at an incredible rate before they are slaughtered for meat. All of them are ending out in our plate, and the concentrates, fertilizers, pesticides and other chemical compounds used on the animals and fruits or veggies will find a way to affect our internal organs, especially the liver. What we think of as natural food is in fact poisoned food. Organic food is really hard to find. However, the main problem of today's nutrition is processed food and its abundance. As this is the most common type of food sold by supermarkets and fast-food chains, it's no wonder that we are so exposed to it. The modern day lifestyle is encouraging the consumption of such food, which is only calorie dense, and it has little to no nutritional value.

The daily schedule involves a very stressful job, with plenty of tasks during the day and strict deadlines, but also no time to have a proper meal. That's why people are eating fast food and all kinds of unhealthy snacks like chips. The result is simply frightening, as more and more people are facing the risk of becoming overweight or have diabetes. But this is just the tip of the iceberg. People are becoming aware of this issue, but they still consume this kind of food, probably because it's the cheapest. They are trying all sorts of diets and meal plans, most of them promising amazing results (but not delivering). You can understand the frustration of trying something incredibly radical, without having the results you expect, or even having catastrophic results that impact your health.

If you are still looking for the solution to obesity and many other medical conditions, look no further! Intermittent fasting may be the healthiest and most sustainable method to lose weight, but also to heal yourself from common illnesses caused by an excess of carbs. Also, it can prevent or even reverse some diseases or conditions. This way of eating has several programs you can try, according to your needs and possibilities. They can all provide the same benefits.

Intermittent fasting is not a way of eating that was invented or discovered recently, as it was practiced by humans for thousands of years. Since food was scarce back then, humans were required to hunt, fish or pick vegetables and fruits in order to survive. They never knew when their next meal was going to be and sometimes it took more than a few days to have the next meal. The prehistoric humans were a lot stronger, faster and more agile than modern-day humans, and this involuntary fasting had something to do with it, but also the quality of the food they had back then, as everything they consumed was natural.

Fasting was a procedure which was practiced for religious purposes for a long time, but nowadays it's starting to become more popular, as more and more people are discovering its benefits. It's better to combine intermittent fasting with physical exercise and the keto diet, to maximize (and also to speed up the occurrence of) its beneficial effects. The 3 of these can form the "health triad" or the "Holy Trinity of a healthy lifestyle." It may sound a bit much, but trust me, after experiencing the benefits of them you will come to see that its reputation is not misplaced. So, what are you waiting for? Go out there are experience the benefits of IF for yourself today!

Bibliography

1. Berardi, John, et al. "All About Intermittent Fasting, Chapter 11." *Precision Nutrition*, www.precisionnutrition.com/intermittent-fasting/appendix-b-tips-and-tricks.

2. Fung, Jason. "Autophagy – a Cure for Many Present-Day Diseases?" *Diet Doctor*, 19 Dec. 2017, www.dietdoctor.com/autophagy-cure-many-present-day-diseases.

3. Fung, Jason, and Andreas Eenfeldt. "Intermittent Fasting for Beginners – The Complete Guide – Diet Doctor." *Diet Doctor*, 21 May 2019, www.dietdoctor.com/intermittent-fasting/.

4. George, Lesley. "Intermittent Fasting And Muscle Gain: Go To Guide To Fasting Like A Pro • Shapezine - Digital Health & Fitness Tracking Blog." *Shapezine - Digital Health & Fitness Tracking Blog*, 10 July 2018, shapescale.com/blog/health/intermittent-fasting-muscle-gain/.

5. Gunnars, Kris. "How Many Calories Should You Eat Per Day to Lose Weight?" *Healthline*, Healthline Media, 6 July 2018, www.healthline.com/nutrition/how-many-calories-per-day#section1.

6. Jarreau, Paige, and Essential Information. "The 5 Stages of Intermittent Fasting." *LIFE Apps | LIVE and LEARN*, 26 Feb. 2019, lifeapps.io/fasting/the-5-stages-of-intermittent-fasting/.

7. Land, S. (2018). *Metabolic autophagy.* Independently Published,

8. Lefave, Samantha. "8 Major Mistakes People Make When Intermittent Fasting." *What's Good by V*, 31 Jan. 2019, whatsgood.vitaminshoppe.com/intermittent-fasting-mistakes/.

9. Levy, Jillian. "Benefits of Autophagy, Plus How to Induce It." *Dr. Axe*, 4 Sept. 2018, draxe.com/benefits-of-autophagy/.

10. Long, Yun Chau, and Juleen R Zierath. "AMP-Activated Protein Kinase Signaling in Metabolic Regulation." *The Journal of Clinical Investigation*, American Society for Clinical Investigation, 3 July 2006, www.ncbi.nlm.nih.gov/pmc/articles/PMC1483147/.

11. Matus, Mizpah. *Alternate Day Diet*, www.freedieting.com/alternate-day-diet.

12. Michal, Anthony. "9 Common Intermittent Fasting Mistakes." *Anthony Mychal*, 26 Oct. 2017, anthonymychal.com/intermittent-fasting-mistakes/

13. "NCI Dictionary of Cancer Terms." *National Cancer Institute*, www.cancer.gov/publications/dictionaries/cancer-terms/def/mtor.

14. Spritzler, Franziska, and Andreas Eenfeldt. "What Is Ketosis? Is It Safe? – Diet Doctor." *Diet Doctor*, 22 Mar. 2019, www.dietdoctor.com/low-carb/ketosis.

15. West, Helen. "How to Fast Safely: 10 Helpful Tips." *Healthline*, Healthline Media, 2 Jan. 2019, www.healthline.com/nutrition/how-to-fast#section1.